MOSBY'S®

Medical-Surgical
Memory Notecards

Visual, Mnemonic and Memory Aids for Nurses

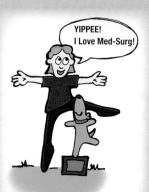

YIPPEE!
I Love Med-Surg!

Jo Ann Zerwekh
EdD, MSN, RN
President/CEO
Nursing Education Consultants, Inc.
Chandler, Arizona

Ashley Garneau
PhD, RN
Nursing Faculty
Department of Nursing
GateWay Community College
Phoenix, Arizona

Tyler Zerwekh
DrPH, MPH, REHS
Senior Manager
Environmental Health and Safety,
    North America Facilities
Luminex Corporation
Austin, Texas

ELSEVIER

T0346188

Elsevier
3251 Riverport Lane
St. Louis, Missouri 63043

MOSBY'S MEDICAL-SURGICAL MEMORY NOTECARDS:
VISUAL, MNEMONIC AND MEMORY AIDS FOR NURSES

ISBN: 978-0-443-26131-2

Content Strategist: Yvonne Alexopoulos, Grace Onderlinde
Content Development Specialist: Deborah Poulson
Publishing Services Manager: Deepthi Unni
Senior Project Manager: Manchu Mohan
Senior Design Direction: Brian Salisbury

Printed in India.

Last digit is the print number: 9 8 7 6 5 4 3 2 1

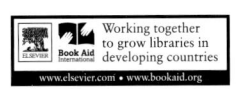

Brittany Bass, DNP, MSN, RN, CNE
Assistant Academic Program Director of Clinical Site Based Learning
Capella University
Minneapolis, Minnesota

Contents

ENDOCRINE, 1

Acromegaly, **2**
Diabetes Insipidus, **4**
Hyperthyroidism, **6**
Hypothyroidism, **8**
Diabetes Mellitus—Type 1 Signs and Symptoms, **10**
Diabetes Mellitus—Type 2, **12**
Blood Glucose Mnemonics, **14**
Methods to Diagnose Diabetes Mellitus, **16**
Triangle of Diabetes Management, **18**
Diabetic Ketoacidosis, **20**
Hyperosmolar-Hyperglycemic State, **22**
Hypoglycemia, **24**
Exercise Guide for Diabetic Fitness, **26**
Metabolic Syndrome, **28**
Addison Disease, **30**
Cushing Syndrome, **32**
Adrenal Gland Hormones, **34**

HEMATOLOGY, 35

Anemia, **36**
Blood Administration, **38**
Acute Blood Transfusion Reactions, **40**
Delayed Blood Transfusion Reactions, **42**
Nursing Management of a Blood Transfusion Reaction, **44**
Hemophilia, **46**
Sickle Cell Crisis, **48**
Symptoms of Leukemia, **50**

RESPIRATORY, 51

Symptoms of Hypoxia, **52**
Asthma, **54**
Pneumonia, **56**

Chronic Obstructive Pulmonary Disease, **58**
Emphysema, **60**
Chronic Bronchitis, **62**
Pulmonary Embolus, **64**
Pulmonary Edema, **66**
Tuberculosis, **68**
Pneumothorax, **70**
Acute Respiratory Distress Syndrome, **72**
Obstructive Sleep Apnea, **74**
COVID-19 Signs and Symptoms, **76**

VASCULAR, 77

Progression of Atherosclerosis, **78**
Hypertension, **80**
Hypertension Nursing Care, **82**
Hypertensive Crisis, **84**
Peripheral Vascular Disease, **86**
Venous Thromboembolism, **88**
Aortic Dissection, **90**
Stages of Shock, **92**

CARDIAC, 93

Chronic Stable Angina, **94**
Myocardial Infarction, **96**
FACES of Heart Failure, **98**
Left-Sided Heart Failure, **100**
Right-Sided Heart Failure, **102**
Treating Heart Failure, **104**

GASTROINTESTINAL, 105

Normal Elimination, **106**
Appendicitis, **108**
Peritonitis, **110**
Bowel Obstruction, **112**
Types of Bowel Obstructions, **114**
Types of Ostomies, **116**

GERD, **118**
Peptic Ulcer Disease, **120**
Crohn's Disease, **122**
Dumping Syndrome, **124**
SIR Hernia, **126**

LIVER, BILIARY, PANCREAS, 127

Cirrhosis: Later Clinical Manifestations, **128**
Hepatic Encephalopathy, **130**
Hepatitis, **132**
Hepatitis A and E, **134**
Cholecystitis, **136**
Laparoscopic Versus Open Cholecystectomy, **138**
Pancreatitis, **140**

NEUROLOGY, 141

Increased Intracranial Pressure, **142**
Increased Intracranial Pressure—Cushing Triad, **144**
Seizures, **146**
Stroke Symptoms, **148**
FAST Recognition of a Stroke, **150**
Left CVA, **152**
Right CVA, **154**
CVA—Functioning VS Affected, **156**
Spinal Cord Injury, **158**
Autonomic Dysreflexia, **160**
Parkinson Disease, **162**
Amyotrophic Lateral Sclerosis, **164**
Multiple Sclerosis, **166**
Guillain-Barré Syndrome, **168**
Myasthenia Gravis, **170**
Cholinergic Crisis, **172**
Bell Palsy, **174**
Migraine Headache Symptoms (POUND), **176**
Tetanus, **178**

MUSCULOSKELETAL, 179

Fracture Classification, **180**
Hip Fracture, **182**
Care of Patient in Traction, **184**
Osteoarthritis, **186**
Rheumatoid Arthritis, **188**
Joint Replacements, **190**
Osteoporosis Risk Factors, **192**
Osteoporosis, **194**
Sprains and Strains—Nursing Care, **196**

REPRODUCTIVE, 197

Menopause, **198**
Post-Mastectomy Nursing Care, **200**
TURP, **202**

URINARY—KIDNEY, 203

Urinary Tract Infection (UTI), **204**
Urinary Calculi, **206**
Acute Kidney Injury (AKI)—Stages, **208**
Acute Kidney Injury (AKI)—Phases, **210**
Chronic Kidney Disease (CKD)—End Stage, **212**
Kidney Transplant Rejection, **214**
Urinary Diversion, **216**

INTEGUMENTARY, 217

Depth of Burns, **218**
Lyme Disease, **220**
Melanoma, **222**
Rocky Mountain Spotted Fever, **224**
Tips on Healing Wounds, **226**

EAR AND EYE, 227

Cataract, **228**
Glaucoma, **230**
Corneal Transplant Surgery, **232**
Causes of Hearing Loss, **234**

IMMUNE, 235

Anaphylactic Reaction, **236**
Systemic Lupus Erythematosus (SLE), **238**
Human Immunodeficiency Virus (HIV) Infection, **240**

EMERGENCY PREPAREDNESS, 241

Types of Disasters, **242**
Disaster Management, **244**
Triage, **246**
Emergency Response Plan, **248**

Index, **249**

ACROMEGALY

* Diagnosis - ↑Plasma Insulin-like Growth Factor (IGF-1)
CT Scan, MRI

Oral Glucose Tolerance Test (OGTT) -
(Glucose Level Does Not Drop)

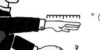

* Clinical Manifestations -

Enlarged Pituitary
- Headaches
- Visual Problems

Facial Changes
- Slanting Forehead
- Coarse Facial Features
- Protruding Jaw
- Thickened Lips

Hypertrophy of Soft Tissue
Menstrual Changes
Enlargement of Small Bones
  in Hands and Feet

What You Need to Know
Acromegaly

DEFINITION

Acromegaly is a rare anterior pituitary disorder caused by the excessive production of growth hormone (GH). It usually occurs because of a benign GH-secreting adenoma and develops after epiphyseal closure. Gigantism is due to excessive GH secretion prior to fusion of epiphyseal growth plates in children and adolescents.

COMPLICATIONS

- Cardiovascular disease
- Diabetes, colorectal cancer
- Sleep apnea, carpal tunnel syndrome

RECOGNIZE AND ANALYZE CUES

- Physical changes occur slowly over many years
- Patient notices an enlarging shoe and ring size

MEDICAL MANAGEMENT: GENERATE SOLUTIONS

- Drugs—octreotide, pasireotide, lanreotide (somatostatin analogs); bromocriptine, cabergoline (dopamine agonists); pegvisomant (GH antagonists)
- Surgery—hypophysectomy (transsphenoidal approach) is treatment of choice
- Radiation therapy—does not have immediate effect

NURSING MANAGEMENT: TAKE ACTION

1. Preoperative—teach about nasal packing and need to breathe through mouth.
2. Monitor neurological status hourly for first 24 hours, then q4h.
3. Monitor "mustache" dressing ("drip" pad) for cerebrospinal fluid (CSF) drainage.
4. Keep the head of the bed elevated at least 30 degrees.
5. Assess nasal drainage for quantity, quality, and the presence of glucose (present in CSF).
6. A light yellow color at the edge of clear drainage on the dressing is called the *halo sign* and indicates CSF.
7. Teach to avoid coughing, sneezing, or blowing nose early after surgery.
8. Teach to use dental floss and nonirritating oral mouth rinses rather than toothbrushing.
9. Observe for complications such as transient diabetes insipidus, CSF leakage, infection, and increased intracranial pressure.

DIABETES INSIPIDUS (DI)

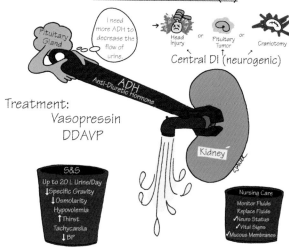

I need more ADH to decrease the flow of urine.

Pituitary Gland

Head Injury   or   Pituitary Tumor   or   Craniotomy

Central DI (neurogenic)

ADH
Anti-Diuretic Hormone

Treatment:
Vasopressin
DDAVP

Kidney

S&S
Up to 20 L Urine/Day
↓Specific Gravity
↓Osmolarity
Hypovolemia
↑Thirst
Tachycardia
↓BP

Nursing Care
Monitor Fluids
Replace Fluids
✓Neuro Status
✓Vital Signs
✓Mucous Membranes

What You Need to Know
Diabetes Insipidus

DEFINITION

Diabetes insipidus (DI) is a posterior pituitary gland problem in which water loss is caused by either an antidiuretic hormone (ADH) deficiency or an inability of the kidneys to respond to ADH. Central (neurogenic) DI is the most common form.

RISK FACTORS

- Trauma/head injury, brain surgery
- Brain tumors, infections (e.g., meningitis, encephalitis)

COMPLICATIONS

- Severe dehydration if patient unable to obtain water can lead to death
- Disturbed electrolyte balance

RECOGNIZE AND ANALYZE CUES

- Polydipsia (excessive thirst), polyuria (2–20 L/day)
- Specific gravity ↓1.005
- ↓Urine osmolarity, ↑serum osmolarity (due to hypernatremia)

MEDICAL MANAGEMENT: GENERATE SOLUTIONS

- Fluid replacement—orally or intravenous (IV) (hypotonic saline or D5W)
- Drugs for central (neurogenic) DI—desmopressin (DDAVP), vasopressin

NURSING MANAGEMENT: TAKE ACTION

1. Monitor for signs of dehydration and electrolyte imbalance.
2. Monitor level of consciousness, vital signs, I&O, daily weights.
3. Make sure patient is not deprived of fluids for more than 4 hours because they cannot reduce urine output and severe dehydration can result.
4. Teach about the need for lifelong drug therapy (permanent DI) and how to assess symptoms, and adjust medication as prescribed for changes in condition (e.g., the onset of polyuria and polydipsia may indicate the need for another dose of medication).

Important nursing interventions	Serious/life-threatening implications
Common signs & symptoms	Patient teaching

HYPERTHYROIDISM

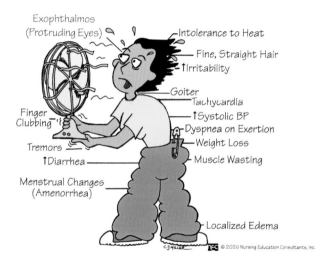

Exophthalmos
(Protruding Eyes)

Intolerance to Heat

Fine, Straight Hair

↑Irritability

Goiter

Tachycardia

↑Systolic BP

Dyspnea on Exertion

Weight Loss

Muscle Wasting

Finger
Clubbing

Tremors

↑Diarrhea

Menstrual Changes
(Amenorrhea)

Localized Edema

© 2026 Nursing Education Consultants, Inc.

What You Need to Know
Hyperthyroidism

DEFINITION

Hyperthyroidism occurs when there is excessive thyroid hormone secretion from the thyroid gland or from the ingestion of synthetic thyroid hormones. The most common form of the disease is Graves disease, an autoimmune disorder that is also called toxic diffuse goiter.

RECOGNIZE AND ANALYZE CUES

- ↑T3 and T4; low or undetectable thyroid-stimulating hormone (TSH) level
- Radioactive iodine uptake: ↑with Graves disease

COMPLICATIONS

- Acute thyrotoxicosis (thyroid storm or thyrotoxic crisis)—monitor for fever (>102°F [38.9°C]), tachycardia, and systolic hypertension

MEDICAL MANAGEMENT: GENERATE SOLUTIONS

- Drugs—antithyroid (propylthiouracil, methimazole)
- Iodine—SSKI or Lugol solution
- Radioactive iodine (RAI) therapy
- Beta-adrenergic blockers (propranolol, atenolol) for thyrotoxicosis
- Total or subtotal thyroidectomy for cases not responding to nonsurgical management

NURSING MANAGEMENT: TAKE ACTION

1. Monitor for relief of signs and symptoms following medical therapy.
2. Do not palpate goiter or thyroid tissue if hyperthyroid symptoms are present.
3. Assess temperature often—an increase of even 1°F (1.8°C) may indicate an impending thyroid crisis, which needs to be reported to the healthcare provider (HCP).
4. Teach the patient with exophthalmos to elevate the head of the bed at night and use artificial tears. If unable to close eyelids, recommend gently taping the lids closed at bedtime to prevent drying of the cornea.
5. Encourage a high-calorie diet with snacks.
6. Promote comfort by lowering the room temperature.
7. Reduce stimulation and encourage rest.
8. Provide preoperative and postoperative care for thyroid surgery, if indicated.
9. Airway obstruction after thyroid surgery is an emergency.
10. Have a tracheostomy tray in patient's room.

HYPOTHYROIDISM

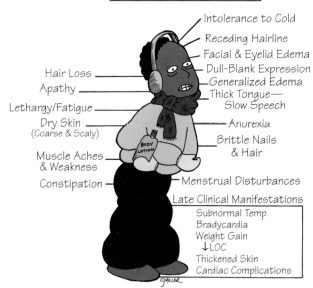

Intolerance to Cold

Receding Hairline

Facial & Eyelid Edema

Dull-Blank Expression

Generalized Edema

Thick Tongue—
Slow Speech

Hair Loss

Apathy

Lethargy/Fatigue

Dry Skin
(Coarse & Scaly)

Anorexia

Brittle Nails
& Hair

Muscle Aches
& Weakness

Constipation

Menstrual Disturbances

Late Clinical Manifestations

Subnormal Temp
Bradycardia
Weight Gain
↓LOC
Thickened Skin
Cardiac Complications

BODY LOTION

Endocrine

What You Need to Know
Hypothyroidism

DEFINITION

Hypothyroidism occurs when there is a deficiency of thyroid hormone secretion from the thyroid gland that slows the metabolic rate.

RISK FACTORS

- Iodine deficiency
- Thyroiditis
- Associated with using medications such as amiodarone and lithium
- Develops posttreatment for hyperthyroidism or RAI therapy

COMPLICATIONS

- Myxedema coma
  - Sluggishness, drowsiness, impairment in consciousness
  - Hypotension, hypoglycemia, hypothermia, hypoventilation
- Death due to respiratory failure and cardiovascular collapse

RECOGNIZE AND ANALYZE CUES

- ↓T3 and T4; ↑TSH level
- ↑Cholesterol and triglycerides
- Goiter (depending on cause of hypothyroidism)

MEDICAL MANAGEMENT: GENERATE SOLUTIONS

- Drugs—levothyroxine

NURSING MANAGEMENT: TAKE ACTION

1. Monitor response to thyroid hormone replacement; advise that it will be about 7 days before they begin to feel better.
2. Monitor vital signs, body weight, activity level, and change in appetite.
3. Assess for cold intolerance, constipation, and signs of depression.
4. Teach the importance of lifelong thyroid hormone therapy.
5. Promote a positive self-image.
6. Assess for myxedema coma.
   - Causes are infection, drugs (opioids, tranquilizers, barbiturates), exposure to cold, and trauma.
7. Observe for the development of heart failure with thyroid hormone replacement.

DIABETES MELLITUS - TYPE 1
SIGNS & SYMPTOMS

Polyuria
↑Urination

Polydipsia
↑Thirst

Polyphagia
↑Hunger

- Weight Loss
- Fatigue
- ↑Frequency of Infections
- Rapid Onset
- Insulin Dependent
- Familial Tendency
- Age of onset <20 years

© 2026 Nursing Education Consultants, Inc.

Endocrine

What You Need to Know
Diabetes Mellitus—Type 1 Signs and Symptoms

DEFINITION

Diabetes mellitus (DM) is a chronic multisystem disease characterized by hyperglycemia due to the absence of—or a severe decrease in—the secretion or utilization of insulin. Type 1 DM is caused by insulin deficiency following pancreatic β-cell destruction, which leads to the inability of the pancreas to make insulin.

RISK FACTORS

- Genetic predisposition
- Viral infection

ACUTE COMPLICATIONS

- Diabetic ketoacidosis (DKA) caused by the absence of insulin and generation of ketoacids
- Hyperglycemic-hyperosmolar state (HHS) caused by insulin deficiency and profound dehydration
- Hypoglycemia from too much insulin or too little glucose

CHRONIC COMPLICATIONS

- Macrovascular—cardiovascular disease, stroke, reduced immunity
- Microvascular—retinopathy, peripheral neuropathy, nephropathy

RECOGNIZE AND ANALYZE CUES

- Classic 3 Ps—polyuria, polydipsia, polyphagia

MEDICAL MANAGEMENT: GENERATE SOLUTIONS

- Drug—insulin
- Diet—carbohydrate counting
- Regular, consistent exercise

NURSING MANAGEMENT: TAKE ACTION

1. ABCs of diabetes to reduce the risk of heart attack and stroke.
   - Control A1c—less than 7%.
   - Blood pressure—keep below 130/80 mm Hg (for most people).
   - Cholesterol—keep low-density lipoprotein (LDL) cholesterol level below 100 mg/dL.
2. Teach how to administer insulin, monitor glucose levels, and manage DM during acute illness and surgery.
3. Teach signs and symptoms of hyperglycemia and hypoglycemia emergencies.
4. Teach about the importance of safe and healthy glucose levels by adequate diet and regular exercise.
5. Encourage wearing a medic alert bracelet.

TYPE 2 DIABETES

Genetic Mutations = Insulin Resistance
& Familial Tendency

- Polyuria
- Polydipsia
- Recurrent Infections
- Visual Changes
- Fatigue, ↓Energy
- HbA1c ↑6.5%, FBS -↑126 mg/dl.
- Prediabetes FBS 100–125 mg/dL
- Metabolic Syndrome

Metabolic Syndrome -
↑Risk for Diabetes

- ↑Triglycerides
- ↓HDL's
- ↑B/P
- Central Obesity
- Sedentary Lifestyle
- FBS > 126 mg/dL
- Most Common ↑35 yrs

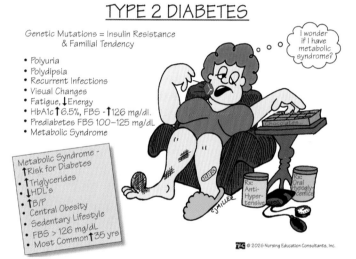

Endocrine

What You Need to Know
Diabetes Mellitus—Type 2

DEFINITION

Type 2 DM is characterized by a combination of inadequate insulin secretion and insulin resistance. The pancreas makes insulin; however, the body does not make enough insulin, does not use it effectively, or both.

RISK FACTORS

- Family history
- Obesity, physical inactivity, metabolic syndrome
- Drug or chemical induced (e.g., glucocorticoids, antiretroviral therapy, immunosuppressants)
- Gestational diabetes or given birth to a newborn weighing over 9 lb

COMPLICATIONS

- DKA caused by the absence of insulin and generation of ketoacids
- HHS caused by insulin deficiency and profound dehydration
- Hypoglycemia from too much insulin or too little glucose

RECOGNIZE AND ANALYZE CUES

- Symptoms of type 2 DM often develop slowly
- Symptoms are often nonspecific

MEDICAL MANAGEMENT: GENERATE SOLUTIONS

- Drugs—oral hypoglycemic agents, noninsulin injectable agents, insulin

NURSING MANAGEMENT: TAKE ACTION

1. Initiate a weight reduction and regular exercise program.
2. ABCs of diabetes to reduce the risk of heart attack and stroke.
    - Control A1c—less than 7%.
    - Blood pressure—keep below 130/80 mm Hg (for most people).
    - Cholesterol—keep LDL cholesterol level below 100.
3. Teach how to administer insulin, monitor glucose levels, and manage DM during acute illness and surgery.
4. Teach signs and symptoms of hyperglycemia and hypoglycemia emergencies.
5. Promote safe and healthy glucose levels by adequate diet and regular exercise.
6. Encourage wearing a medic alert bracelet.

Important nursing interventions	Serious/life-threatening implications
Common signs & symptoms	Patient teaching

BLOOD GLUCOSE MNEMONIC

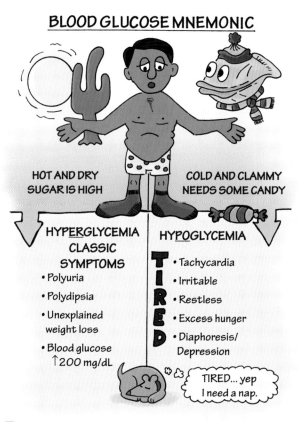

HOT AND DRY
SUGAR IS HIGH

COLD AND CLAMMY
NEEDS SOME CANDY

**HYPERGLYCEMIA
CLASSIC
SYMPTOMS**
- Polyuria
- Polydipsia
- Unexplained
  weight loss
- Blood glucose
  ↑200 mg/dL

HYPOGLYCEMIA

T
I • Tachycardia
R • Irritable
E • Restless
D • Excess hunger
  • Diaphoresis/
  Depression

TIRED... yep
I need a nap.

What You Need to Know

Blood Glucose Mnemonics

DEFINITION

Blood glucose is the amount of glucose or sugar in the blood. Glucose is a major source of energy for most cells of the body, including brain cells. Glucose is a simple sugar (a monosaccharide) that comes primarily from ingesting food. Glucose levels are elevated after eating. Insulin, which is made in the beta cells of the pancreatic islets of Langerhans, is secreted in response to the increased glucose level.

RECOGNIZE AND ANALYZE CUES

- Hyperglycemia—increased level of glucose
- Hypoglycemia—decreased level of glucose
  Use mnemonics to help you and patients with DM to remember the symptoms and treatment when blood glucose is high or low.

MEDICATIONS AFFECTING GLUCOSE LEVELS

- Drugs that *increase* levels of glucose—antidepressants (tricyclics), antipsychotics, beta-adrenergic blocking agents, corticosteroids, cyclosporins, IV dextrose infusion, dextrothyroxine, diazoxide, diuretics, epinephrine, estrogens, glucagon, isoniazid, lithium, niacin, phenothiazines, phenytoin, salicylates (acute toxicity), triamterene, and statins
- Drugs that *decrease* levels of glucose—acetaminophen, alcohol, alpha-glucosidase inhibitors, anabolic steroids, biguanides, clofibrate, disopyramide, gemfibrozil, incretin mimetics, insulin, monoamine oxidase inhibitors, meglitinides, pentamidine, propranolol, sulfonylureas, and thiazolidinediones

NURSING MANAGEMENT: TAKE ACTION

1. Evaluate blood glucose levels according to the time of day they are obtained. Levels increase after meals.
2. Blood glucose assessment must be performed frequently in new patients with DM to determine appropriate insulin or oral hypoglycemic therapy.
3. Stress can cause increased serum glucose levels, along with caffeine.
4. Many females who are pregnant may experience some degree of glucose intolerance, which may result in gestational diabetes.
5. Remember that many drugs affect glucose levels.

METHODS TO DIAGNOSE DIABETES MELLITUS

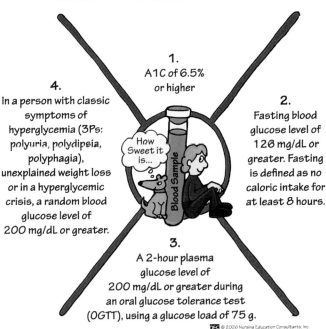

1.
A1C of 6.5% or higher

4.
In a person with classic symptoms of hyperglycemia (3Ps: polyuria, polydipsia, polyphagia), unexplained weight loss or in a hyperglycemic crisis, a random blood glucose level of 200 mg/dL or greater.

2.
Fasting blood glucose level of 128 mg/dL or greater. Fasting is defined as no caloric intake for at least 8 hours.

3.
A 2-hour plasma glucose level of 200 mg/dL or greater during an oral glucose tolerance test (OGTT), using a glucose load of 75 g.

How Sweet it is...

Blood Sample

© 2026 Nursing Education Consultants, Inc.

What You Need to Know
Methods to Diagnose Diabetes Mellitus

DEFINITION

The diagnosis of DM is confirmed using one of four methods. Methods 1 through 3 require repeat testing for a confirming diagnosis. If there are obvious symptoms of the classic 3 Ps (polyuria, polyphagia, polydipsia) with a random blood glucose level of $\geq 200\,mg/dL$, repeat testing is not needed.

FACTORS AFFECTING RESULTS

- False-positive or increased value results can be due to:
  - Severe carbohydrate dietary restriction
  - Acute illness
  - Medications (e.g., contraceptives, corticosteroids)
  - Restricted activity, bed rest, immobility
- False-negative results can be due to:
  - Impaired gastrointestinal (GI) absorption
  - Recent ingestion of acetaminophen

NURSING MANAGEMENT: TAKE ACTION

1. Teach client that the A1C measures the amount of glycosylated hemoglobin (Hgb) as a percentage of total Hgb. For example, an A1C of 5.5% means that 5.5% of the total Hgb has glucose attached to it. The glucose stays attached to the red blood cell for the life of the cell (about 120 days).
   - A1C provides an average measure of glucose levels over the previous 2 to 3 months.
   - A1C does *not* consider fluctuations in glucose and hence is *not* a good indicator of how often the patient has a high or low glucose level.
   - Fasting is *not* needed to collect an A1C sample.
2. Teach patients to have an A1C regularly monitored with the goal of it being less than 7.0%. Emphasize that when the A1C is maintained at near-normal levels, the risk of developing microvascular and macrovascular complications is significantly reduced.
3. Be sure to provide patient preparation for the specific test ordered.

Important nursing interventions	Serious/life-threatening implications
Common signs & symptoms	Patient teaching

TRIANGLE OF DIABETIC MANAGEMENT

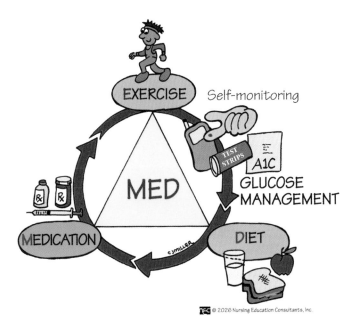

Self-monitoring

GLUCOSE MANAGEMENT

© 2026 Nursing Education Consultants, Inc.

=========== **What You Need to Know** ===========

Triangle of Diabetes Management

DEFINITION

Management of DM involves diet interventions, a planned exercise program, and drugs to lower blood glucose levels. Think of the mnemonic MED—medication, exercise, diet. Blood glucose monitoring is an integral part of the triangle of DM management.

NURSING MANAGEMENT: TAKE ACTION

1. Medication
   - Type 1 DM requires insulin; type 2 DM may require antidiabetic drugs and in some cases insulin.
   - Encourage self-monitoring of blood glucose.
   - Teach patients with DM that keeping blood glucose levels within prescribed target ranges can prevent or delay complications.
2. Exercise
   - Teach to exercise 150 minutes/week (30 minutes, 5 days/week) moderate intensity aerobic activity (e.g., walking briskly, golfing, dancing).
   - Should perform resistance training 2–3 times/week, unless contraindicated.
   - Exercise lowers glucose levels, and hypoglycemia can occur up to 48 hours after the activity.
   - Should be taught to monitor glucose levels before, during, and after exercise.
3. Diet
   - Teach to choose healthy food choices that are low in saturated and trans fat.
   - Focus on diet sources, such as vegetables, fruits, whole grains, legumes, and dairy products.
   - Should limit regular soda, fruit juices, and alcohol.
   - Encourage eating meals at regular times and intervals.

Important nursing interventions	Serious/life-threatening implications
Common signs & symptoms	Patient teaching

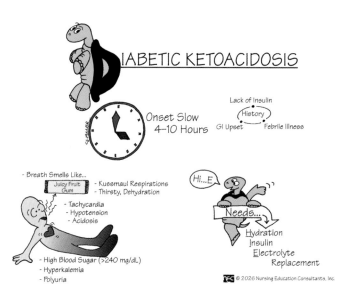

DIABETIC KETOACIDOSIS

Onset Slow
4–10 Hours

Lack of Insulin

History

GI Upset — Febrile Illness

- Breath Smells Like...
  Juicy Fruit Gum
  - Kussmaul Respirations
  - Thirsty, Dehydration
  - Tachycardia
  - Hypotension
  - Acidosis

- High Blood Sugar (>240 mg/dL)
- Hyperkalemia
- Polyuria

Hi...E

Needs...

Hydration
Insulin
Electrolyte
  Replacement

© 2026 Nursing Education Consultants, Inc.

What You Need to Know
Diabetic Ketoacidosis

DEFINITION

Diabetic ketoacidosis (DKA) is a complication of diabetes characterized by uncontrolled hyperglycemia, metabolic acidosis, and increased production of ketones.

RISK FACTORS

- Infection, illness
- Inadequate insulin dose
- Other stressors

COMPLICATIONS

- Hypovolemia, acidosis, kidney failure
- Death, if condition not treated

RECOGNIZE AND ANALYZE CUES

- Polyuria, polydipsia, polyphagia
- Rotting citrus fruit odor to the breath, vomiting, abdominal pain
- Glucosuria, ketonuria, serum glucose >250 mg/dL
- Dehydration, tachycardia, weakness, confusion, shock, and coma

MEDICAL MANAGEMENT: GENERATE SOLUTIONS

- Fluid resuscitation with 0.9% normal saline to treat dehydration
- Continuous regular IV insulin
- Administer potassium to correct hypokalemia
- Administer sodium bicarbonate to correct acidosis

NURSING MANAGEMENT: TAKE ACTION

1. Assess airway, level of consciousness, hydration status, electrolytes, and serum glucose.
   - Monitor hypotonic IV fluids and continuous IV regular insulin.
   - Administer 5% dextrose in 0.45% normal saline when serum glucose levels reach 250 mg/dL to prevent hypoglycemia and cerebral edema—can occur when serum osmolarity declines too rapidly.
   - Subcutaneous (subQ) insulin started when the patient can take oral fluids and ketosis has resolved.
2. Monitor carefully to prevent rapid drops in serum glucose to avoid cerebral edema.
3. Teach about consulting with the diabetes HCP when these problems occur to prevent DKA:
   - Blood glucose exceeds 250 mg/dL and does not respond to therapy.
   - Ketonuria lasts for more than 24 hours.
   - Cannot take food or fluids.
   - An illness lasts more than 1 to 2 days.

HYPEROSMOLAR HYPERGLYCEMIC STATE (HHS)

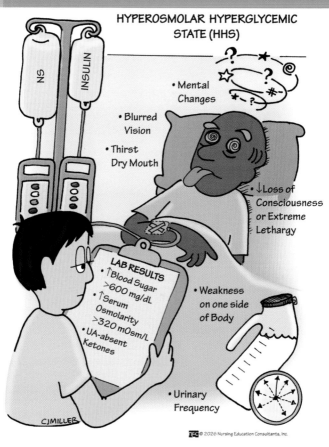

NS

INSULIN

- Mental Changes
- Blurred Vision
- Thirst Dry Mouth
- ↓Loss of Consciousness or Extreme Lethargy

LAB RESULTS
- ↑Blood Sugar >600 mg/dL
- ↑Serum Osmolarity >320 mOsm/L
- UA-absent Ketones

- Weakness on one side of Body
- Urinary Frequency

CJMILLER

© 2026 Nursing Education Consultants, Inc.

Endocrine

What You Need to Know

Hyperosmolar-Hyperglycemic State

DEFINITION

Hyperglycemic-hyperosmolar state (HHS) is a hyperosmolar (increased blood osmolarity) state caused by hyperglycemia that occurs more often in older adults with type 2 DM of which many are unaware that they are experiencing HHS. HHS results from sustained osmotic diuresis leading to extremely high blood glucose levels and is less common than DKA. HHS differs from DKA in that ketone levels are absent or low, and blood glucose levels are very high.

RISK FACTORS

- Urinary tract infections
- Pneumonia, sepsis, acute illness

COMPLICATIONS

- Hypovolemia, acidosis, kidney failure
- Death, if condition not treated

RECOGNIZE AND ANALYZE CUES

- Onset of symptoms is slow
- Symptoms may resemble a stroke
  - Coma occurring with serum osmolarity >320 mOsm/L
- ↑Serum glucose >600 mg/dL, ↑serum osmolarity >320 mOsm/L
- Ketones are absent or minimal in both blood and urine
- Dehydration or electrolyte loss is the same as for DKA

MEDICAL MANAGEMENT: GENERATE SOLUTIONS

- A medical emergency with high mortality rate
- Fluid replacement with normal saline to increase blood volume is a priority

NURSING MANAGEMENT: TAKE ACTION

1. Assess airway, level of consciousness, hydration status, electrolytes, and serum glucose.
   - Monitor hypotonic IV fluids and continuous IV regular insulin.
   - Administer 5% dextrose in 0.45% normal saline when serum glucose levels reach 250 mg/dL to prevent hypoglycemia and cerebral edema, which can occur when serum osmolarity declines too rapidly.
   - SubQ insulin started when the patient can take oral fluids and ketosis has resolved.
2. Monitor carefully to prevent rapid drops in serum glucose to avoid cerebral edema.
3. Assess for signs of cerebral edema (e.g., abrupt change in mental status, abnormal neurologic signs, coma).

Important nursing interventions	Serious/life-threatening implications
Common signs & symptoms	Patient teaching

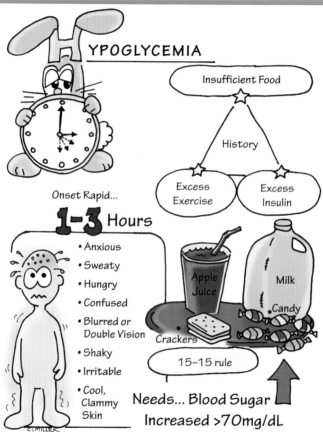

HYPOGLYCEMIA

Insufficient Food

History

Excess Exercise

Excess Insulin

Onset Rapid...

1-3 Hours

- Anxious
- Sweaty
- Hungry
- Confused
- Blurred or Double Vision
- Shaky
- Irritable
- Cool, Clammy Skin

Apple Juice

Milk

Candy

Crackers

15-15 rule

Needs... Blood Sugar Increased >70mg/dL

CJ MILLER

=== **What You Need to Know** ===

Hypoglycemia

DEFINITION

Hypoglycemia is a low blood glucose level. Glucose level falls below 70 mg/dL.

RISK FACTORS

- Hypoglycemia unawareness (no warning signs low blood sugar)—occurs with a long-standing history of diabetes.
- Excess insulin compared with food intake and physical activity.
- Insulin injected at the wrong time (when it is peaking) relative to exercise.
- Decreased food intake resulting from missed or delayed meals.
- Decreased glucose production in the liver after alcohol ingestion.
- Reduced insulin clearance due to progressive kidney failure.

RECOGNIZE AND ANALYZE CUES

- Cool, clammy, sweaty, confusion, headache
- Weakness, double or blurred vision, palpitations, seizures, coma

MEDICAL MANAGEMENT: GENERATE SOLUTIONS

- Hospitalized patient—20–50 mL of 50% dextrose IV
- Hospitalized patient—follow the 15–15 rule if patient is conscious
- Glucagon 1 mg intramuscularly (deltoid)

NURSING MANAGEMENT: TAKE ACTION

1. "15–15 Rule"
   - Give 15 g of simple, fast-acting carbohydrate (CHO), such as 4–6 oz of orange juice (apple juice for patients with diabetes), 6–10 pieces of hard candy, 1 T of honey, 3 graham crackers, or glucose tablets if the blood glucose level is less than 70 mg/dL (or 30 g if less than 50 mg/dL). Recheck glucose in 15 minutes.
   - If they can swallow, give a liquid form of CHO, although any fast-acting CHO source can be used.
   - Avoid foods that are high in fiber or fat (e.g., chocolate) because it slow down the absorption of glucose.
   - If the blood glucose recheck within 15 minutes is still low, the same treatment is given again.
   - If unable to swallow, an IV dose of concentrated dextrose or subQ glucagon is indicated.
2. Instruct to ingest alcohol only with or shortly after eating a meal with enough CHO to prevent hypoglycemia.

EXERCISE GUIDE FOR
DIABETIC **FIT**NESS

F Frequency
Regular (5 days/week)

I Intensity
60%–80% Of Maximal Heart Rate

T Time
Aerobic Activity
30 Minutes/5 Days/Week
Total: 150 Min./Wk
With 5 Min.
Warm Up & Cool Down

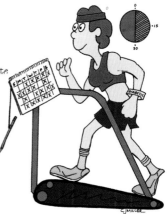

CJMILLER

—————————————— **What You Need to Know** ——————————————
Exercise Guide for Diabetic Fitness

DEFINITION

Regular, consistent exercise is an essential part of DM and prediabetes management because it improves carbohydrate metabolism and insulin sensitivity. Increased physical activity and weight loss reduce the risk of type 2 DM in patients with prediabetes.

NURSING MANAGEMENT: TAKE ACTION

1. Exercise needs to be consistent; does not have to be vigorous to be effective (e.g., brisk walking).
2. Encourage exercise activities that are enjoyable to promote consistency.
3. Teach to use properly fitting footwear to avoid rubbing or injury to the feet.
4. Teach the importance of a warm-up period and a cool-down period and to begin gradually and increase slowly.
5. Teach to stay hydrated while exercising; do not exercise in extreme hot or cold environments.
6. Encourage carrying a simple sugar to eat during exercise if symptoms of hypoglycemia occur.
7. Stress the importance of when to exercise—best done after meals when the glucose level is rising. Avoid exercising within 1 hour of insulin injection or near time of peak insulin action.
8. Teach the importance of monitoring glucose levels before, during, and after exercise.
9. Before exercise, if glucose level is ≤100 mg/dL, teach to eat a 15-g CHO snack. After 15–30 minutes of exercise, recheck glucose level. Delay exercise if blood glucose is <100 mg/dL. Encourage talking to the HCP about lowering medication dose(s) if hypoglycemia occurs consistently.
10. Those with type 1 DM should only engage in vigorous exercise when blood glucose levels are 100 to 250 mg/dL.
11. Teach that exercise-induced hypoglycemia may occur several hours after completing exercise.
    - Explain the importance of remembering that extra CHO and less insulin may be needed during the 24-hour period following exercise because the glucose-lowering effects of exercise can last up to 48 hours after the activity.

METABOLIC SYNDROME - SYNDROME X

Avoid the X Factor
Leads to: Diabetes, Stroke,
and Heart Disease.

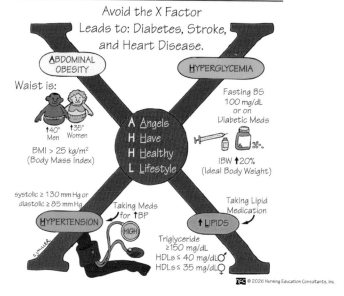

ABDOMINAL OBESITY

Waist is:

↑40" Men   ↑35" Women

BMI > 25 kg/m²
(Body Mass Index)

HYPERGLYCEMIA

Fasting BS
100 mg/dL
or on
Diabetic Meds

IBW ↑20%
(Ideal Body Weight)

A Angels
H Have
H Healthy
L Lifestyle

systolic ≥ 130 mm Hg or
diastolic ≥ 85 mm Hg

HYPERTENSION

Taking Meds
for ↑BP
HIGH

Taking Lipid
Medication

↑LIPIDS

Triglyceride
≥150 mg/dL
HDLs ≤ 40 mg/dL♂
HDLs ≤ 35 mg/dL♀

What You Need to Know
Metabolic Syndrome

DEFINITION

Metabolic syndrome, also called insulin resistance syndrome or syndrome X, is a cluster of conditions that increase the risk factors for type 2 DM, stroke, and cardiovascular disease (CVD). It is closely linked to being overweight or obese and inactive, and it is also linked to insulin resistance.

RISK FACTORS

- Increased age
- Ethnicity (increased in Hispanic females)
- Obesity, diabetes, sleep apnea
- Nonalcoholic fatty liver disease
- Polycystic ovary syndrome

COMPLICATIONS

- Type 2 DM, stroke, CVD

RECOGNIZE AND ANALYZE CUES

- Features of the syndrome include:
  - Waist circumference of ≥40 inches (102 cm) for males and ≥35 inches (89 cm) for females
  - Hyperglycemia: fasting blood glucose level of ≥100 mg/dL or receiving drug treatment for ↑glucose level
  - Hypertension: systolic ≥130 mm Hg or diastolic ≥85 mm Hg or on drug treatment for hypertension
  - Triglyceride level ≥150 mg/dL or on drug treatment for ↑triglycerides
  - High-density lipoprotein cholesterol ≤40 mg/dL for males or ≤50 mg/dL for females
- Diagnosed if there are three of the five features listed above.

MEDICAL MANAGEMENT: GENERATE SOLUTIONS

- Management is aimed at reducing the risks of obesity, managing hypertension, and preventing complications.

NURSING MANAGEMENT: TAKE ACTION

1. Teach the importance of a healthy lifestyle to prevent metabolic syndrome.
   - Exercising at least 30 minutes on most days.
   - Eating plenty of vegetables, fruits, lean protein, and whole grains.
   - Limiting saturated fat and salt in the diet.
   - Maintaining a healthy weight; weight loss program.
   - Not smoking.

ADDISON DISEASE
Adrenocortical Insufficiency

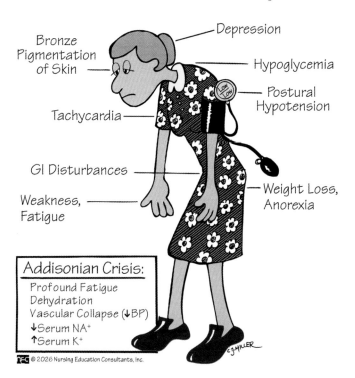

Depression

Bronze Pigmentation of Skin

Hypoglycemia

Postural Hypotension

Tachycardia

GI Disturbances

Weakness, Fatigue

Weight Loss, Anorexia

Addisonian Crisis:
Profound Fatigue
Dehydration
Vascular Collapse (↓BP)
↓Serum NA⁺
↑Serum K⁺

© 2026 Nursing Education Consultants, Inc.

=== **What You Need to Know** ===
Addison Disease

DEFINITION

Addison disease (also known as primary adrenal insufficiency or hypoadrenalism) is an uncommon disorder of the adrenal glands. Most cases are caused by an autoimmune response where the adrenal cortex is destroyed by antibodies.

RISK FACTORS

- Familial
- Other autoimmune disorders (e.g., type 1 DM, thyroid disease, pernicious anemia, celiac disease)

COMPLICATIONS

- Addisonian or adrenal crisis is a life-threatening complication

RECOGNIZE AND ANALYZE CUES

- Weakness, fatigue, postural hypotension
- GI upset—abdominal pain, chronic diarrhea
- Salt craving, weight loss, depression
- Hypoglycemia, hyperkalemia, hyponatremia
- Bronzing skin pigmentation, vitiligo
- Diagnosis: adrenocorticotropic hormone (ACTH) simulation test—absent or no increase in cortisol level

MEDICAL MANAGEMENT: GENERATE SOLUTIONS

- Lifelong hormone therapy
  - Glucocorticoids—prednisone, hydrocortisone
  - Mineralocorticoids—fludrocortisone
- Diet changes—increased salt in diet

NURSING MANAGEMENT: TAKE ACTION

1. Monitor for fluid deficit and hyperkalemia; prevent hypoglycemia.
   - Obtain daily weight when hospitalized; I&O.
   - Monitor for signs and symptoms of addisonian crisis.
2. Teach about lifelong medication therapy.
   - Teach the importance of increased dosages of corticosteroids during stressful situations (e.g., surgery, fever, tooth extraction, illness).
   - Explain the signs and symptoms of corticosteroid deficiency and excess (Cushing syndrome).
   - Encourage wearing a medic alert bracelet.

Important nursing interventions	Serious/life-threatening implications
Common signs & symptoms	Patient teaching

CUSHING SYNDROME
Corticosteroid Excess

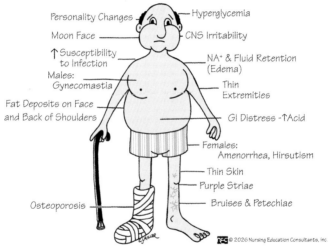

Personality Changes

Moon Face

↑Susceptibility to Infection

Males: Gynecomastia

Fat Deposits on Face and Back of Shoulders

Osteoporosis

Hyperglycemia

CNS Irritability

NA⁺ & Fluid Retention (Edema)

Thin Extremities

GI Distress -↑Acid

Females: Amenorrhea, Hirsutism

Thin Skin

Purple Striae

Bruises & Petechiae

© 2026 Nursing Education Consultants, Inc.

--- **What You Need to Know** ---

Cushing Syndrome

DEFINITION

Cushing syndrome or hypercortisolism is a clinical condition that results from chronic exposure to excess corticosteroids, especially glucocorticoids, or from the excess secretion of cortisol from the adrenal cortex.

RISK FACTORS

- Secretion of hormone due to tumor or hyperplasia
- Taking ACTH or glucocorticoids in treating asthma, organ transplant, cancer chemotherapy

COMPLICATIONS

- Osteoporosis, hypertension
- Type 2 DM, serious infections

RECOGNIZE AND ANALYZE CUES

- Moon face, buffalo hump, truncal obesity
- Hypertension, hyperglycemia, hypervolemia
- Hypokalemia, hypernatremia
- Diagnosis: dexamethasone suppression test

MEDICAL MANAGEMENT: GENERATE SOLUTIONS

- Normalize hormone secretion; possible gradual tapering of corticosteroid therapy
- Adrenalectomy if there is an adrenal tumor or hyperplasia
- Drugs (poor candidate for surgery)—ketoconazole and mitotane to reduce cortisol secretion; mifepristone to control hyperglycemia

NURSING MANAGEMENT: TAKE ACTION

1. Monitor for fluid overload; I&O.
2. Assess for infection.
3. Provide emotional support as related to changes in appearance.
4. Encourage wearing a medic alert bracelet.
5. Teach about the condition and how to manage it.
6. Provide preoperative and postoperative care.
   - Assess for postoperative bleeding due to vascularity of adrenal glands.
   - Anticipate high doses of corticosteroids during and after surgery.

ADRENAL GLAND HORMONES

S Sugar (Glucocorticoids)

S Salt (Mineralcorticoids)

S Sex (Androgens)

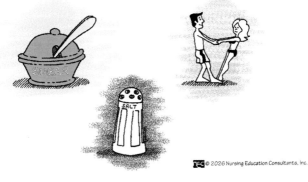

====== **What You Need to Know** ======
Adrenal Gland Hormones

DEFINITION

The adrenal glands are small vascular organs that are located on the top of each kidney. The adrenal gland consists of two parts—the adrenal cortex and the adrenal medulla. The adrenal cortex and medulla function like two separate but interrelated glands. The adrenal cortex secretes glucocorticoids, mineralocorticoids, and sex hormones. The adrenal medulla secretes the catecholamines (e.g., epinephrine, norepinephrine, and dopamine), which act as both neurotransmitters when secreted by neurons and hormones when secreted by the adrenal medulla. They are part of the "fight or flight" sympathetic nervous system response.

ADRENAL CORTEX

1. Glucocorticoids
   - Cortisol is the main glucocorticoid produced by the adrenal cortex and is essential to life.
   - Secreted in a diurnal pattern (rises during the day; declines in the evening).
   - Has anti-inflammatory, immunosuppressive, and growth-suppressing effects and is released under stress conditions.
   - Regulates blood glucose; CHO, protein, and fat metabolism; sodium and water balance.
   - When you hear the term *corticosteroid*, it refers to both *glucocorticoids* and *mineralocorticoids*.
2. Mineralocorticoids
   - Aldosterone is the most potent of the naturally occurring mineralocorticoids and maintains extracellular fluid volume.
   - Acts to promote sodium and water reabsorption and potassium excretion in the kidney.
   - Hyperkalemia, hyponatremia, and angiotensin II stimulate the production of aldosterone.
3. Sex hormones
   - Secretes small amounts of estrogen and androgens in both sexes.
   - Adrenal secretion of these hormones is usually not significant because the gonads (ovaries and testes) secrete much larger amounts of estrogens and androgens.
   - The most common adrenal androgens are dehydroepiandrosterone and androstenedione.
   - In females, the adrenal gland is the major source of androgens.

ADRENAL MEDULLA

1. Epinephrine
   - Major hormone secreted by the adrenal medulla.
   - Can activate alpha1, alpha2, beta1, and beta2 receptors.
2. Norepinephrine
   - Can activate alpha1, alpha2, and beta1 receptors.
3. Dopamine
   - Can activate dopamine, beta1, and, at high doses, alpha1 receptors.

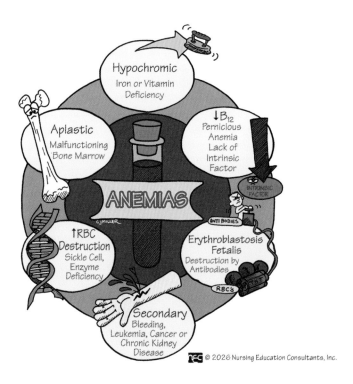

ANEMIAS

Hypochromic
Iron or Vitamin
Deficiency

Aplastic
Malfunctioning
Bone Marrow

↓B₁₂
Pernicious
Anemia
Lack of
Intrinsic
Factor

↑RBC
Destruction
Sickle Cell,
Enzyme
Deficiency

Erythroblastosis
Fetalis
Destruction by
Antibodies

Secondary
Bleeding,
Leukemia, Cancer or
Chronic Kidney
Disease

=== **What You Need to Know** ===
Anemia

DEFINITION

Anemia is a deficiency in the number of red blood cells (RBCs) or a decrease in the quality or quantity of hemoglobin (Hgb) and/or volume of packed RBCs (hematocrit). It is not a specific disease but a clinical indicator due to (1) blood loss (acute or chronic), (2) impaired RBC production, (3) increased RBC destruction, or (4) a combination of these factors.

COMPLICATIONS

- Cardiac dysrhythmias, heart failure, myocardial infarction
- Hypoxia, life-threatening complications

RECOGNIZE AND ANALYZE CUES

- Pallor, cool to touch, brittle nails (chronic), jaundice
- Tachycardia, murmurs, gallops, orthostatic hypotension
- Dyspnea on exertion, $\downarrow SpO_2$
- Fatigue, increased need for sleep, low energy level
- Diagnostics: males, Hgb level of <13.5 g/dL; females, Hgb <12.0 g/dL indicate anemia

MEDICAL MANAGEMENT: GENERATE SOLUTIONS

- Treat underlying cause of the anemia
- Iron deficiency anemia—iron supplement, diet therapy
- Vitamin B_{12} deficiency anemia—B_{12} injections (weekly, then monthly), diet therapy
- Folic acid deficiency anemia—folic acid supplement
- Aplastic anemia—blood transfusion, immunosuppressive therapy, hematopoietic stem cell transplant (HSCT)
- Sickle cell crisis—oxygen, hydration, opioid analgesic, hydroxyurea, Endari

NURSING MANAGEMENT: TAKE ACTION

1. Anticipate blood transfusions, drug therapy (e.g., iron supplements, opioid analgesics), and oxygen therapy.
2. Encourage rest and arrange activity periods according to energy levels.
   - Teach the patient to avoid activity right after meals to reduce O_2 consumption.
   - Assist the patient when doing regular activities (e.g., ambulation, transfers, personal care) to minimize fatigue.
3. Monitor the patient's cardiorespiratory response to activity (e.g., tachycardia, dysrhythmias, dyspnea, diaphoresis, pallor, tachypnea).
4. Teach about diet and lifestyle changes related to the specific type of anemia as this can reverse some of the symptoms.

BLOOD ADMINISTRATION

* Determine Patient's
- Allergies
- Previous Transfusion Reactions

Filter →

* Administer Within 30 Minutes of Receiving From Blood Bank

* Never Add **ANY** Meds to Blood Products

KEY POINTS

- Verify Patient's ID
- Check the HCP's Order
- Check labels on blood bag & blood bank transfusion record
- Baseline vitals - (Then per policy)
- #18G or #20G gauge needle
- Normal saline IV solution
- Blood administration set with filter
- Severe reactions most likely first 15 minutes & first 50 mL
- Blood tubing should be changed after 4 hours

* Check Crossmatch Record With
  <u>2</u> Nurses:
- ABO-Group
- RH Type
- Patient's Name
- ID Blood Band
- Hospital #
- Expiration Date

* Do **NOT** Warm Unless Risk of Hypothermic Response **THEN** Only By Specific Blood Warming Equipment

* Infuse Each Unit Over 2–4 Hours **BUT** No Longer Than 4 Hours

© 2026 Nursing Education Consultants, Inc.

What You Need to Know
Blood Administration

DEFINITION

A blood transfusion is a procedure in which donated whole blood or blood components (e.g., platelets, plasma) are collected from one person (the donor) and transfused into the bloodstream of another person (the recipient).

COMPLICATIONS

- Transfusion reaction

MEDICAL MANAGEMENT: GENERATE SOLUTIONS

- Need a healthcare provider (HCP) order or prescription to administer blood or blood components.
- Obtain a type and crossmatch blood specimen.

NURSING MANAGEMENT: TAKE ACTION

1. Before transfusion nursing responsibilities
   - Initiate an intravenous (IV) access with normal saline using a blood administration set, Y-tubing set-up with blood filter (about 170 μm to remove sediment from stored blood product).
   - With another registered nurse, verify the patient by name and number, check blood compatibility, and note expiration time. *Remember human error is the most common cause of incompatibility reactions.*
2. During transfusion nursing responsibilities
   - Begin infusion slowly. *Remain with the patient for the first 15 to 30 minutes.*
   - Severe reactions usually occur with the infusion of the first 50 mL of blood.
   - Monitor vital signs (VS) q15 minutes; if no reaction, take VS hourly.
   - Never add medications to blood products because they may clot the blood during the transfusion.
3. After transfusion nursing responsibilities
   - After transfusion is completed, discontinue the blood infusion, switch to the normal saline line, dispose of the bag and tubing according to agency and blood bank policies.
   - Document all aspects of the transfusion and patient's response.

Important nursing interventions	Serious/life-threatening implications
Common signs & symptoms	Patient teaching

ACUTE BLOOD TRANSFUSION REACTIONS

ALLERGIC ANAPHYLACTIC
- History of Allergies
- Onset Immediate or Up to 24 hours
- Mild (Allergic)
- Severe (Anaphylactic)— Life Threatening

FEBRILE
- Is Nonhemolytic
- Often Received Multiple Transfusions
- Sensitized to Donor WBCs

HEMOLYTIC
- Incompatible Blood Administered
- Occurs Immediately
- Life Threatening

SEPTIC
- Contaminated Blood Product Administered
- Onset Is Rapid (Bacterial)

TRALI
- Life Threatening
- Rapid Onset (1–6 hours)
- Pulmonary Symptoms

TACO
- Blood Infused Too Quickly
- Pulmonary Symptoms
- Older Adult

What You Need to Know
Acute Blood Transfusion Reactions

DEFINITION

An acute reaction to a blood transfusion that can range in severity from mild to life threatening.

RECOGNIZE AND ANALYZE CUES

1. Allergic (anaphylactic)
   - Allergic (mild): flushing, itching, hives
   - Anaphylactic: anxiety, abdominal pain, hives, dyspnea, wheezing, progressing to bronchospasm, ↓blood pressure (BP), shock, cardiac arrest
2. Febrile
   - Sudden chills, rigors, fever
   - Headache, vomiting
   - Tachypnea, ↑heart rate (HR), ↓BP
3. Hemolytic
   - Develops in first 15 minutes; may occur up to 2 hours after
   - Fever with or without chills
   - Back, abdominal, chest, or flank pain
   - Dyspnea, tachypnea, ↑HR, ↓BP
   - Hemoglobinuria, bleeding
   - Acute jaundice, dark urine
   - Sense of impending doom "something is wrong"
   - Acute kidney injury, shock, cardiac arrest, disseminated intravascular coagulation (DIC), death
4. Septic
   - Rapid onset of chills, rigors, fever
   - Vomiting, diarrhea, ↑HR, ↓BP, shock
5. Transfusion-related acute lung injury (TRALI)
   - Rapid onset of dyspnea within 1 to 6 hours
   - Fever, chills, hypotension
   - Tachypnea, dyspnea, hypoxemia, respiratory failure
   - Noncardiogenic pulmonary edema, frothy sputum
6. Transfusion-associated circulatory overload (TACO)
   - Hypertension, bounding pulse, ↑HR
   - Distended jugular veins
   - Dyspnea, pulmonary congestion
   - Restlessness, headache
   - Confusion

MEDICAL MANAGEMENT: GENERATE SOLUTIONS

- See Nursing Management of Blood Transfusion Reaction notecard for the medical management (page 43)

NURSING MANAGEMENT: TAKE ACTION

- See Nursing Management of Blood Transfusion Reaction notecard (page 43)

TYPES OF DELAYED TRANSFUSION REACTIONS

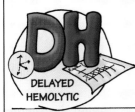

DELAYED HEMOLYTIC

- Occurs Within 3 Days or Months Later
- Hemolysis of Transfused RBCs
- Fever
- Jaundice
- Increased Bilirubin
- Decreased Hemoglobin

- Rare Condition
- Life Threatening
- Occurs in Immunosuppressed
- Pancytopenia
- Rash, Fever
- Diarrhea, Vomiting
- Chronic Hepatitis
- Recurrent Infection

TA-GVHD

TRANSFUSION ASSOCIATED GRAFT-VS-HOST

DISEASE

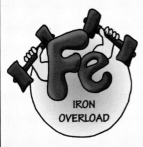

IRON OVERLOAD

- Excess Iron Deposited in Heart, Liver, Pancreas, Joints
- Occurs With Numerous Transfusions >20
- Heart Failure, Dysrhythmias
- Impaired Thyroid & Gonadal Function
- Diabetes
- Arthritis
- Cirrhosis, Liver Failure

Hematology

What You Need to Know

Delayed Blood Transfusion Reactions

DEFINITION

Delayed transfusion reactions include delayed hemolytic reactions, transfusion-associated graft-versus-host disease (TA-GVHD), and iron overload.

RECOGNIZE AND ANALYZE CUES

- Delayed hemolytic reaction
  - Occurs within 3 days or months later
  - Hemolysis of transfused RBCs
  - Fever
  - Jaundice
  - ↑Serum bilirubin
  - ↓Hgb
- TA-GVHD
  - Rare condition, life threatening
  - Occurs in immunosuppressed patients
  - Pancytopenia, rash, fever
  - Diarrhea, vomiting
  - Chronic hepatitis
  - Recurrent infection
- Iron overload
  - Excess iron deposited in heart, liver, pancreas, joints
  - Occurs with numerous transfusions >20
  - Heart failure, dysrhythmias
  - Impaired thyroid and gonadal function
  - Diabetes, arthritis
  - Cirrhosis, liver failure

MEDICAL MANAGEMENT: GENERATE SOLUTIONS

- Delayed hemolytic reaction
  - Drugs: eculizumab, rituximab, prednisone
  - IV immunoglobulin therapy
- TA-GVHD
  - Irradiation of blood products to reduce the risk of donor lymphocytes attacking an immunocompromised patient
- Iron overload
  - Drugs: deferoxamine, deferasirox, deferiprone (chelating agents)
  - Phlebotomy

NURSING MANAGEMENT: TAKE ACTION

1. Monitor patients and provide supportive care.
2. Anticipate end-of-life care as often a delayed transfusion reaction can lead to death.

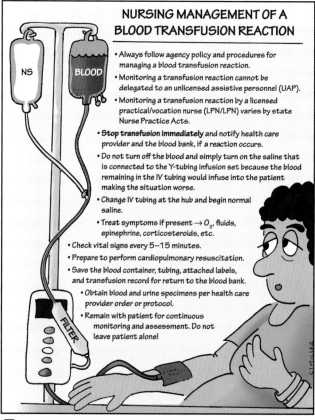

NURSING MANAGEMENT OF A BLOOD TRANSFUSION REACTION

- Always follow agency policy and procedures for managing a blood transfusion reaction.
- Monitoring a transfusion reaction cannot be delegated to an unlicensed assistive personnel (UAP).
- Monitoring a transfusion reaction by a licensed practical/vocation nurse (LPN/LPN) varies by state Nurse Practice Acts.
- **Stop transfusion immediately** and notify health care provider and the blood bank, if a reaction occurs.
- Do not turn off the blood and simply turn on the saline that is connected to the Y-tubing infusion set because the blood remaining in the IV tubing would infuse into the patient making the situation worse.
- Change IV tubing at the hub and begin normal saline.
- Treat symptoms if present → O_2, fluids, epinephrine, corticosteroids, etc.
- Check vital signs every 5–15 minutes.
- Prepare to perform cardiopulmonary resuscitation.
- Save the blood container, tubing, attached labels, and transfusion record for return to the blood bank.
- Obtain blood and urine specimens per health care provider order or protocol.
- Remain with patient for continuous monitoring and assessment. Do not leave patient alone!

What You Need to Know
Nursing Management of a Blood Transfusion Reaction

NURSING MANAGEMENT: TAKE ACTION

1. Acute hemolytic
   - Monitor VS; maintain BP with IV fluids.
   - Change IV tubing at the hub; administer normal saline to maintain patent IV access.
   - Treat shock and DIC if present.
   - Obtain blood and urine samples; send specimens to the laboratory.
   - Give diuretics as prescribed to maintain urine flow.
   - Insert an indwelling urinary catheter; monitor hourly urine output.
   - Anticipate dialysis if kidney failure occurs.
2. Febrile (nonhemolytic)
   - Administer antipyretics to treat fever.
   - Anticipate leukocyte-reduced blood products being prescribed.
   - Administer acetaminophen or diphenhydramine 30 minutes before transfusion.
   - Do not restart transfusion unless there is an HCP order.
3. Allergic
   - Administer antihistamine, corticosteroid, and epinephrine.
   - If symptoms are mild and transient (no fever, dyspnea, or wheezing), transfusion may be restarted slowly with HCP's order.
   - Do not restart transfusion if fever or pulmonary symptoms develop.
4. Anaphylactic
   - Monitor VS frequently; provide O_2.
   - Administer epinephrine, antihistamines, corticosteroids, and $\beta2$ agonists.
   - Start CPR, if indicated.
   - Do not restart transfusion.
5. Septic (bacterial contamination)
   - Monitor VS; provide O_2.
   - Obtain the culture of patient's blood.
   - Anticipate that other tests may be ordered to discern from a hemolytic reaction.
   - Treat septicemia—antibiotics, IV fluids, vasopressors.
6. TRALI
   - Monitor VS frequently; provide O_2.
   - Administer corticosteroids and vasopressors.
   - Start CPR if needed; provide ventilatory and BP support.
   - Draw blood for arterial blood gases and HLA or antileukocyte antibodies and other tests to discern hemolysis or circulatory overload.
   - Obtain chest x-ray.
7. TACO
   - Monitor VS; provide O_2; administer diuretics.
   - Position upright (high Fowler) with feet in dependent position.
   - Obtain chest x-ray if ordered.

HEMOPHILIA

(Inherited Blood Disorder
Factor VIII, Classic, or Type A)

- Avoid Injury

- No Cure

- Avoid Meds That
  ↑Bleeding
  ASA **NO** NSAIDS

- Good Nutrition

- Good Dental
  Hygiene

- IV Administration
  Of Deficient
  Clotting
  Factor

Slow, Persistent, Prolonged
Bleeding from Minor Trauma/Cuts

Prolonged Nosebleeds

Bruises Easily

Warm, Painful, Swollen Joints
(Hemathrosis)

GI Bleeding

COFFEE-GROUND EMESIS

Hematuria

TARRY STOOLS

© 2026 Nursing Education Consultants, Inc.

What You Need to Know
Hemophilia

DEFINITION

Hemophilia is an X-linked recessive genetic disorder caused by a defective or deficient co-agulation factor. There are two major types of hemophilia, distinguishable only by laboratory tests: hemophilia A (classic hemophilia, factor VIII deficiency) and hemophilia B (Christmas disease, factor IX deficiency). Hemophilia A is more common.

RISK FACTORS

- Genetic inheritance pattern
  - Female carriers transmit the genetic defect to 50% of their sons; 50% of their daughters are carriers.
  - Males with hemophilia do not transmit the genetic defect to their sons, but all their daughters are carriers.
  - While rare, female hemophilia can occur in offspring of a male with hemophilia and a female carrier. (*This is because males with hemophilia are living longer due to improved treatment.*)

COMPLICATIONS

- Hemarthrosis; internal bleeding into the brain
- Airway obstruction from neck or pharynx bleeding

RECOGNIZE AND ANALYZE CUES

- Bleeding episodes that can become life threatening

MEDICAL MANAGEMENT: GENERATE SOLUTIONS

- Factor replacement—during active bleeding episodes and as prophylaxis
- Desmopressin (DDAVP)—used to treat mild cases
- Aminocaproic acid and tranexamic acid—antifibrinolytic agents used to prevent recurrent bleeding episodes

NURSING MANAGEMENT: TAKE ACTION

1. Initiate immediate measures to control bleeding.
   - Apply direct pressure or ice, pack the area with fibrin foam; apply topical hemostatic agents (e.g., thrombin).
   - Administer the specific coagulation factor.
   - Monitor joint bleeding—in addition to giving replacement factors, use the "RICE" protocol—**r**est, **i**ce, **c**ompress/wrap joint, **e**levate.
2. Anticipate any life-threatening complications.
3. Teach the patient to wear a Medic Alert bracelet.

Important nursing interventions	Serious/life-threatening implications
Common signs & symptoms	Patient teaching

SICKLE CELL CRISIS
(Inherited Red Blood Cell Disorder)

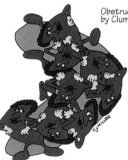

Obstruction of Vessels
by Clumped Sickled Cells

Vasoocclusive Crisis
- Pain
  Acute Abdominal
  Hand/Foot Syndrome
- Splenic Atrophy due to
  Repeated Scarring
- Stroke (Cerebral Infarction)
- Kidney — Ischemia

Aplastic Crisis
- Suppression of RBCs
  due to Infection

RBC Destruction
Acute Chest Syndrome
Fever
Cough
↑ Respiratory & Heart
Rate Hypoxia

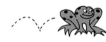

HOP -
Hydration and Electrolytes
Oxygen—Bed Rest to ↓ O_2 needs
Pain Relief

What You Need to Know
Sickle Cell Crisis

DEFINITION

Sickle cell disease is a group of inherited, autosomal recessive disorders characterized by an abnormal form of Hgb (Hgb S) in the RBCs. Sickle cell crisis is a severe, painful, acute exacerbation of RBC sickling, causing a vaso-occlusive crisis.

RISK FACTORS

- Dehydration, hypoxia, infection

COMPLICATIONS

- Infection (pneumonia), sepsis
- Acute chest syndrome (tissue infarction, fat embolism)
- Multiple organ dysfunction syndrome

RECOGNIZE AND ANALYZE CUES

- Pain due to poor perfusion and impaired gas exchange due to RBC clumping

MEDICAL MANAGEMENT: GENERATE SOLUTIONS

- Drugs: opioid analgesics, hydroxyurea, Endari, crizanlizumab
- Oxygen therapy; hydration (IV or oral)

NURSING MANAGEMENT: TAKE ACTION

1. Administer pain medication.
2. Maintain adequate hydration (limit caffeine); IV fluids.
3. Avoid taking BP with a standard or automatic external arm cuff.
4. Monitor pulse oximetry, peripheral pulses, capillary refill q1h.
5. Prevent infection; promote hand hygiene.
6. Teach patients ways to avoid sickle cell crisis.
   - Drink 3–4 L of fluids daily.
   - Avoid alcoholic drinks and smoking.
   - Avoid hot and cold temperature extremes.
   - Keep extremities warm with socks and gloves.
   - Avoid small airplanes that are not pressurized.
   - Avoid traveling to areas at high altitudes.
   - Avoid strenuous physical exercise; focus on mild, low-impact exercise three times a week when not in crisis.

Important nursing interventions	Serious/life-threatening implications
Common signs & symptoms	Patient teaching

SYMPTOMS OF LEUKEMIA

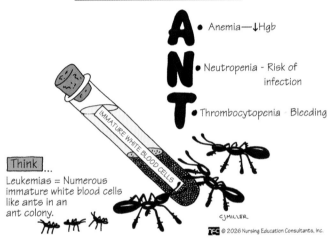

- Anemia—↓Hgb
- Neutropenia - Risk of infection
- Thrombocytopenia · Bleeding

Think ...
Leukemias = Numerous
immature white blood cells
like ants in an
ant colony.

CJMILLER

NEC © 2026 Nursing Education Consultants, Inc.

What You Need to Know
Symptoms of Leukemia

DEFINITION

Leukemia is an uncontrolled proliferation of abnormal white blood cells, which leads to eventual cellular destruction as a result of the infiltration of the leukemic cells into the body tissue. Leukemia occurs in all age groups and is an actual blood cancer that Is classified by cell type: acute myeloid leukemia (AML), acute lymphocytic leukemia (ALL)—most common in children—chronic myelogenous leukemia (CML), and chronic lymphocytic leukemia (CLL).

RISK FACTORS

- Ionizing radiation, viral infection, exposure to chemicals and drugs, genetic and immunity factors

RECOGNIZE AND ANALYZE CUES

- Anemia, fever (infection), and bleeding tendencies occur together
- Anorexia, weight loss, cough, fatigue, lethargy
- Central nervous system involvement: headache, confusion, increased irritability
- Petechiae, bruises easily, epistaxis
- Bone and joint pain; hepatomegaly and splenomegaly

MEDICAL MANAGEMENT: GENERATE SOLUTIONS

- Drugs: corticosteroids, antineoplastic agents
- Hematopoietic stem cell transplant (HSCT)
- Radiation therapy

NURSING MANAGEMENT: TAKE ACTION

1. Monitor temperature—an elevation of even 1°F (0.5°C) above the patient's baseline needs to be reported.
2. Prevent infection—neutropenic precautions; protective environment for HSCT patients.
3. Teach patients ways to prevent infection and stop bleeding.
4. Discourage pets (e.g., fish, birds, cats), fresh flowers, and houseplants because of the possibility of bacteria and virus transmission.
5. Teach patients measures to conserve energy and that shortness of breath and palpitations are symptoms of overactivity.
6. Prevent or limit bleeding episodes.
7. Monitor for adverse effects of chemotherapy and radiation therapy.

HYPOXIA

ASSESSMENT

- Arterial Blood Gases
- Pulmonary Function Studies
- Hemoglobin & Hematocrit
- History
- Pulse Oximetry ↓90%
- Clinical Signs & Symptoms

RISK FACTORS

- Anemia
- Asthma
- Bronchitis
- COPD
- Congenital heart defects
- Emphysema
- Heart Failure
- Pneumonia

Inadequate amount of oxygen available for cellular metabolism

CLINICAL SIGNS & SYMPTOMS

EARLY

- Restless
- Tachycardia
- Dyspnea
- ↑ Agitation
- Diaphoresis
- Retrations
- Altered Level of Conciousness- Confusion, Anxiety

LATE

- ↑ Restlessness
- Somnolence
- Stupor
- Dyspnea
- ↓ Respirations
- Bradycardia
- Cyanosis

Out of Order

KIDS

- Nares Flaring
- Grunting
- Stridor
- Feeding Problems

CJMILLER

What You Need to Know
Symptoms of Hypoxia

DEFINITION

Hypoxia is a condition characterized by an inadequate amount of O_2 available for cellular metabolism.

RISK FACTORS

- Respiratory obstruction and alveolar hypoventilation (chronic obstructive pulmonary disease [COPD], cystic fibrosis, cancer)
- Inadequate circulation due to shock or heart failure
- Inflammatory problems (pneumonia, bronchitis)
- Anemia precipitates hypoxia due to inadequate red blood cell production or deficient or abnormal hemoglobin

COMPLICATIONS

- Acute: respiratory failure, cardiac decompensation, progression to chronic hypoxia
- Chronic: CO_2 narcosis (increase in CO_2 content of blood), cor pulmonale (right-sided heart failure due to respiratory NOT cardiac causes), heart failure

RECOGNIZE AND ANALYZE CUES

- *Early symptoms*: restlessness, tachycardia, tachypnea, exertional dyspnea, orthopnea, tripod positioning, anxiety, difficulty speaking, poor judgment, confusion, disorientation
- *Late symptoms*: extreme restlessness to stupor, severe dyspnea, slowing of respiratory rate, bradycardia, cyanosis (peripheral or central), intercostal retractions

MEDICAL MANAGEMENT: GENERATE SOLUTIONS

- Oxygen therapy
- Additional treatment depends on the underlying problem

NURSING MANAGEMENT: TAKE ACTION

1. Assess the patency of the airway (first/highest priority) and position the patient to maintain a patent airway.
   - Unconscious: position on the side with the chin extended.
   - Conscious: elevate the head of the bed and may position on the side as well, or in a "tripod position" (leaning forward with mouth open).
2. Initiate O_2 if dyspnea is present.
3. Encourage coughing and deep breathing.
4. Suction as needed and as indicated by the amount of sputum and ability to cough.
5. Maintain adequate fluid intake to keep secretions liquefied.
6. Encourage exercises and ambulation as indicated by the condition.
7. Remember … increasing anxiety will accelerate dyspnea if the patient is experiencing severe difficulty breathing.

ASTHMA
(Reactive Airway Disease)

- Triggers
  - Hypersensitivity
  - URI
  - Exercise
  - Air Pollutants
  - Respiratory Infections
  - GERD

- Familial
  Tendency

- Intermittent Reversible
  Airway Obstruction

- Hypoxemia:
  Tachycardia
  ↑ Restlessness
  Tachypnea

Asthma Attack
- Cough
- ↑ Mucus
- Shortness of
  Breath
- Chest Tightness
- Early - ↓$Paco_2$
- Late - ↑$Paco_2$
- Wheezing
  & Prolonged
  Expiration
- Retractions

Emergency:
If symptoms do not
respond to usual treatment
in 30 minutes, patient should
seek medical attention.

Status Asthmaticus
Can be life threatening!

Asthma

DEFINITION

Asthma is an intermittent, reversible obstructive airway problem. It is characterized by exacerbations and remissions. It is a common disorder of childhood but may also cause problems throughout adult life.

RISK FACTORS OR TRIGGERS

- Hypersensitivity (allergens) and airway inflammation
- Air pollutants, tobacco smoke, and occupational factors
- Exercise-induced asthma

COMPLICATIONS

- Attack can be life threatening
- Status asthmaticus

RECOGNIZE AND ANALYZE CUES

- Wheezing, cough, dyspnea, and chest tightness after exposure to a risk factor or trigger
- Symptoms worse at night
- Decreased or absent breath sounds ("silent chest") is an ominous sign

MEDICAL MANAGEMENT: GENERATE SOLUTIONS

- Drugs: inhaled, IV, or oral corticosteroids; inhaled β2-adrenergic agonists; inhaled anticholinergics
- Controller medications: used every day for regular maintenance:
  - Inhaled corticosteroids (ICS); essential to reduce the risk of death and severe exacerbations
  - Long-acting β-agonist (LABA) (formoterol, salmeterol)
- Using ICS-formoterol is preferred (short-acting β2-adrenergic agonists [SABAs] are no longer first-line therapy)
- Reliever (rescue medication) for as-needed relief of breakthrough symptoms
  - SABA—albuterol/levalbuterol
  - Low-dose ICS taken whenever SABA is taken
- Supplemental O_2 to maintain SpO_2 at 90%

NURSING MANAGEMENT: TAKE ACTION

1. Prevent and control asthma episodes.
   - Position for comfort: usually high-Fowler position or tripod position.
   - Monitor response to O_2 therapy, SpO_2 levels, changes in respiratory status.
   - Assess response to bronchodilators and inhalation therapy.
   - Monitor ability to take PO fluids; risk for aspiration is increased.
   - Observe for sudden increase or decrease in restlessness.
   - Assess for side effects of medications, such as tremors and tachycardia.
2. Provide self-management education with a personal asthma action plan developed by healthcare provider (HCP) and patient.

PNEUMONIA

- Obstruction of Bronchioles
- ↓Gas Exchange
- ↑Exudate

Symptoms...

- Cough
- Fever
- Chills
- Tachycardia
- Tachypnea
- Dyspnea
- Pleural Pain
- Malaise
- Respiratory Distress
- ↓Breath Sounds

"I should wear a mask if I am within three feet of the patient."

Droplet Precautions

Cough
Cough

Sputum Specimen

- Productive Cough: Yellow, Bloodstreaked, Rusty Sputum = Infection
- Opportunistic: Pneumocystis jiroveci pneumonia (PCP) Mycobacterium avium complex (MAC)

Drs Orders For Diagnosis
- Sputum Culture
- Chest X-ray
- ABG's

© 2026 Nursing Education Consultants, Inc.

What You Need to Know
Pneumonia

DEFINITION

Pneumonia is an acute inflammatory process caused by a microbial agent; it involves lung parenchyma, including the small airways and alveoli. It can be caused by bacteria, viruses, fungi, or other organisms.

RISK FACTORS

- Chronic upper respiratory tract infection, prolonged immobility
- Smoking and secondhand smoke, decreased immunity (disease and/or age)
- Aspiration of foreign material or gastric contents
- Chronic health problems: cardiac, pulmonary, diabetes, cancer, stroke
- Lack of pneumococcal vaccination
- Nosocomial pneumonia: caused by tracheal intubation, intestinal/gastric tube feedings, ventilator-associated pneumonia

COMPLICATIONS

- Airway obstruction, respiratory failure
- Empyema, sepsis

RECOGNIZE AND ANALYZE CUES

- Fever, chills, tachycardia, tachypnea, dyspnea
- Productive cough: thick, blood-streaked, yellow, purulent sputum
- Pleuritic chest pain, malaise, altered mental status

MEDICAL MANAGEMENT: GENERATE SOLUTIONS

- Drugs: antibiotics, bronchodilators, antivirals, pneumococcal vaccine
- Inhalation therapy: Cool O_2 mist, incentive spirometer
- Chest physiotherapy—suctioning, percussion, and postural drainage

NURSING MANAGEMENT: TAKE ACTION

1. Have the patient turn, cough, and deep breathe.
2. Liquefy secretions; cool mist inhalation.
3. Maintain adequate hydration; administer PO fluids cautiously to prevent aspiration.
4. Evaluate breath sounds and changes in sputum.
5. Monitor SpO_2 and maintain at 95% or above.
6. Position for comfort or place in a semi-Fowler position.

Important nursing interventions	Serious/life-threatening implications
Common signs & symptoms	Patient teaching

COPD

"EMPHYSEMA AND CHRONIC BRONCHITIS"

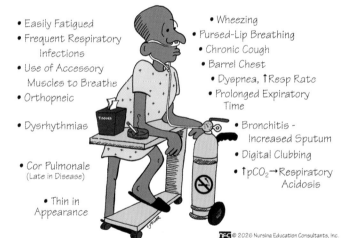

- Easily Fatigued
- Frequent Respiratory Infections
- Use of Accessory Muscles to Breathe
- Orthopneic

- Dysrhythmias

- Cor Pulmonale (Late in Disease)

- Thin in Appearance

- Wheezing
- Pursed-Lip Breathing
- Chronic Cough
- Barrel Chest
- Dyspnea, ↑Resp Rate
- Prolonged Expiratory Time

- Bronchitis - Increased Sputum
- Digital Clubbing
- ↑pCO_2→Respiratory Acidosis

© 2026 Nursing Education Consultants, Inc.

What You Need to Know
Chronic Obstructive Pulmonary Disease

DEFINITION

COPD is a group of chronic lower airway disorders characterized by obstruction of airflow, primarily chronic bronchitis and emphysema. Although each of the disorders (chronic bronchitis, emphysema) may occur individually, it is more common for two or more problems to coexist and the symptoms to overlap.

RISK FACTORS

- Cigarette smoking (including passive smoking)—most common risk factor
- Chronic infections
- Inhaled irritants (from occupational exposure and air pollution)
- Asthma (*asthma-COPD overlap syndrome*)
- Alpha$_1$-antitrypsin deficiency: enzyme deficiency leading to decreased lung elasticity and COPD at an early age (30–45 years)
- Aging: changes in thoracic cage and respiratory muscles and loss of elastic recoil

COMPLICATIONS

- Hypoxemia, acidosis, acute respiratory failure
- Pulmonary hypertension, cor pulmonale (right-sided heart failure)
- Infections (pneumonia)
- Peptic ulcer and gastroesophageal reflux

RECOGNIZE AND ANALYZE CUES

- Symptoms develop slowly

MEDICAL MANAGEMENT: GENERATE SOLUTIONS

- Oxygen therapy to keep SpO$_2$ greater than 90%
- Drugs: bronchodilators (β2-adrenergic agonists, anticholinergics), inhaled corticosteroids (ICS)
- Short-acting β2-adrenergic agonist (SABA)—mainstay of COPD treatment
- Lung transplantation

NURSING MANAGEMENT: TAKE ACTION

1. Teach pursed-lip breathing: inhale through the nose and exhale against pursed lips.
2. Avoid activities that increase dyspnea.
3. Initiate humidified O$_2$ (low flow via nasal cannula or Venturi mask at a rate of 2–4 L/min); should be used when patients experience exertional or resting hypoxemia.
   - Monitor for hypercapnia, hypoxia, and acidosis.
   - Significant increase in PaO$_2$ may decrease respiratory drive (O$_2$ toxicity).
4. Promote a regular exercise program as part of pulmonary rehabilitation.

Important nursing interventions	Serious/life-threatening implications
Common signs & symptoms	Patient teaching

EMPHYSEMA
"PINK PUFFER"

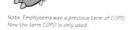

* Alveolar (diffusion) Problem
* ↑CO_2 Retention (Pink)
* Minimal Cyanosis
* Pursed-Lip Breathing
* Dyspnea/↑Resp Rate
* Hyperresonance on Chest Percussion
* Orthopneic
* Barrel Chest
* Exertional Dyspnea
* Prolonged Expiratory Time
* Speaks in Short Jerky Sentences
* Anxious
* Use of Accessory Muscles to Breathe
* Thin appearance

Note: Emphysema was a previous term of COPD. Now the term COPD is only used.

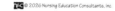

What You Need to Know
Emphysema

DEFINITION

Emphysema is a problem with the alveoli characterized by a loss of alveolar elasticity, overdistention, and destruction, with severe impairment of gas exchange across the alveolar membrane.

RISK FACTORS

- Cigarette smoking (including passive smoking)—most common risk factor
- Chronic infections
- Inhaled irritants (from occupational exposure and air pollution)

COMPLICATIONS

- Bullae in the lungs, pneumothorax
- Cor pulmonale occurs late in disease

RECOGNIZE AND ANALYZE CUES

- Cough is not common, sensation of air hunger
- Use of accessory muscles of respiration, decreased breath sounds
- Anorexia with weight loss, thin in appearance, barrel chest
- No cardiac enlargement; decreased PaO_2 with activity
- Characteristic tripod position—leaning forward with arms braced on knees

MEDICAL MANAGEMENT: GENERATE SOLUTIONS

- Oxygen therapy to keep SpO_2 greater than 90%
- Drugs: bronchodilators (β2-adrenergic agonists, anticholinergics), inhaled corticosteroids (ICS)
- Lung volume reduction surgery

NURSING MANAGEMENT: TAKE ACTION

1. Teach pursed-lip breathing: inhale through the nose and exhale against pursed lips.
2. Avoid activities that increase dyspnea.
3. Administer humidified O_2 (low flow via nasal cannula at a rate of 2–4 L/min).
4. Balance activities and dyspnea.
5. Encourage soft, high-protein, high-calorie, moderate-carbohydrate diet.

Important nursing interventions	Serious/life-threatening implications
Common signs & symptoms	Patient teaching

CHRONIC BRONCHITIS
"BLUE BLOATER"

* Airway Flow Problem
* Color Dusky to Cyanotic
* Recurrent Cough &
  ↑Sputum Production
* Hypoxia
* Hypercapnia ($\uparrow pCO_2$)
* Respiratory Acidosis
* ↑Hgb
* ↑Resp Rate
* Exertional Dyspnea
* ↑Incidence in Smokers
* Digital Clubbing

* Cardiac Enlargement
* Use of Accessory Muscles
  to Breathe
* Leads to Right-Sided Heart Failure: Bilateral Pedal Edema, ↑JVD

Note: Chronic bronchitis was a previous term of COPD.
Now the term COPD is only used.

What You Need to Know
Chronic Bronchitis

DEFINITION

Chronic bronchitis is characterized by an excess secretion of thick, tenacious mucus that decreases ciliary function, interferes with airflow, and causes inflammatory damage to the bronchial mucosa.

RISK FACTORS

- Cigarette smoking (including passive smoking)—most common risk factor
- Chronic infections
- Inhaled irritants (from occupational exposure and air pollution)

COMPLICATIONS

- Respiratory infections
- Polycythemia because of the low PaO_2

RECOGNIZE AND ANALYZE CUES

- Excessive, chronic sputum production (generally not discolored unless infection is present)
- Impaired ventilation, resulting in $\downarrow PaO_2$ and symptoms of hypoxia; $\uparrow PaCO_2$ (CO_2 narcosis)
- Productive cough, exercise intolerance, wheezing, and shortness of breath, progressing to cyanosis
- Dependent edema
- Generally normal weight or overweight
- Cardiac enlargement with cor pulmonale

MEDICAL MANAGEMENT: GENERATE SOLUTIONS

- Oxygen therapy to keep SpO_2 greater than 90%
- Drugs: bronchodilators (β2-adrenergic agonists, anticholinergics), inhaled corticosteroids (ICS)
- Pulmonary rehabilitation

NURSING MANAGEMENT: TAKE ACTION

1. Elevate head of the bed.
2. Monitor for signs of respiratory infection.
3. Teach the patient to increase fluid intake (2–3 L/day) and eat small frequent meals when dyspneic.
4. Teach the patient to avoid dairy products if these increase sputum production.
5. Teach effective coughing and deep-breathing techniques.
6. Administer bronchodilators, ICS medications.

Important nursing interventions	Serious/life-threatening implications
Common signs & symptoms	Patient teaching

PULMONARY EMBOLUS

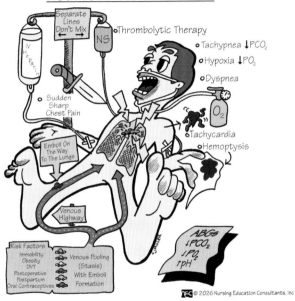

Separate Lines Don't Mix ←→

IV Heparin

NS

Thrombolytic Therapy

Tachypnea ↓PCO_2

Hypoxia ↓PO_2

Dyspnea

Sudden Sharp Chest Pain

O_2

Tachycardia

Hemoptysis

Emboli On The Way To The Lungs

Venous Highway

Risk Factors
Immobility
Obesity
DVT
Postoperative
Postpartum
Oral Contraceptives

Venous Pooling (Stasis) With Emboli Formation

ABGs
↓PCO_2
↓PO_2
↑pH

================ **What You Need to Know** ================
Pulmonary Embolus

DEFINITION

A pulmonary embolism (PE) is an obstruction of a pulmonary artery, most often the result of an embolism caused by a blood clot (thrombus), air, fat, amniotic fluid, bone marrow, or sepsis. The severity of the problem depends on the size of the embolus.

RISK FACTORS

- Venous thromboembolism (VTE)
- Older age, obesity, prolonged immobilization
- Surgery (total hip and knee, hip fracture cancer), joint replacement
- Spinal cord injury, major trauma injury, active cancer
- Hormonal replacement therapy, pregnancy/postpartum, oral contraceptives
- Clotting disorders

COMPLICATIONS

- Pulmonary infarction, pulmonary hypertension
- Death

RECOGNIZE AND ANALYZE CUES

- Dyspnea, pleuritic chest pain, and hemoptysis
- Diagnostics: D-dimer test ↑, enhanced spiral computed tomography (CT) scan, ventilation-perfusion (V/Q) lung scan, arterial blood gases (ABGs)

MEDICAL MANAGEMENT: GENERATE SOLUTIONS

- Respiratory support: O_2, ventilator
- Drugs: anticoagulants (low-molecular-weight heparin, heparin, factor Xa inhibitors, thrombin inhibitors, warfarin, thrombolytics)
- Surgery: embolectomy or insertion of inferior vena cava filter

NURSING MANAGEMENT: TAKE ACTION

1. Identify patients at increased risk; prevent and/or decrease venous stasis (VS).
2. Bed rest and semi-Fowler position, initially.
3. Administer medications—low-molecular-weight heparin recommended for acute PE.
4. Monitor VS, SpO_2, and the effects of oxygen therapy.
5. Monitor laboratory results (platelets, INR, aPTT, etc.).
6. Teach about anticoagulant therapy (continues for at least 3 months).

Important nursing interventions	Serious/life-threatening implications
Common signs & symptoms	Patient teaching

PULMONARY EDEMA

M Meds ➜ Dobutamine, Morphine
A Airway
D Decrease Preload (Nitroglycerin IV)

D Diuretics (Furosemide)
O Oxygen
G Blood Gases (ABGs)

─── **What You Need to Know** ───
Pulmonary Edema

DEFINITION

Pulmonary is caused by an abnormal accumulation of fluid in the lung in both the interstitial and alveolar spaces.

RISK FACTORS

- Left-sided heart failure—most common cause
- Acute respiratory distress syndrome (ARDS)
- Aspiration, inhaled toxins, inflammation (e.g., pneumonia), severe hypoxia, near-drowning
- Anaphylactic (allergic) reaction
- Nephrotic syndrome, liver disease, nutritional disorders
- Non-Hodgkin lymphoma
- Overhydration with IV fluids
- O_2 toxicity

COMPLICATIONS

- Life-threatening medical emergency

RECOGNIZE AND ANALYZE CUES

- Dyspnea, diaphoresis, and wheezing
- Blood-tinged, frothy sputum
- Cool, moist skin
- Tachycardia, S3, S4 gallop, dependent edema

MEDICAL MANAGEMENT: GENERATE SOLUTIONS

- MAD DOG acronym

NURSING MANAGEMENT: TAKE ACTION

1. Place in high-Fowler position with legs dependent.
2. Administer high levels of O_2—5 to 12 L/min with a facemask or 6 to 10 L/min with a nonrebreathing mask with reservoir.
3. Monitor SpO_2 and keep above 90%.
4. May administer noninvasive ventilation (e.g., bilevel positive airway pressure [BiPAP]) or mechanical ventilation.
5. Pulmonary edema is one of the few circumstances of respiratory distress where IV morphine may be given.
6. Ongoing monitoring VS, breathing pattern, breath sounds, urinary output, electrolyte balance, and response to treatment.

TUBERCULOSIS

- Progressive Fatigue
- Malaise
- Anorexia
- Weight Loss

Cough, Cough

- Chronic Cough (Productive)

- Night Sweats
- Hemoptysis (Advanced State)

- Pleuritic Chest Pain

- Low-grade Fever

Tissue

Treatment:	Diagnosis:
TB Medications for 6 Mos or Longer	TB Skin Test (screening)
Decreased Activity	Chest X-Ray
Resp Isolation Until Negative Sputum	Sputum Studies
Frequently Outpatient Treatment	(3 specimens collected on different days)

Tuberculosis

DEFINITION

Tuberculosis (TB) is a reportable communicable disease caused by infection with the bacteria *Mycobacterium tuberculosis*. It usually involves the lungs but can infect any organ, including the brain, kidneys, and bones. *Latent TB infection* occurs in patients who do not have active TB disease and have a positive skin test but are asymptomatic. They cannot transmit the TB bacteria to others but can develop active TB disease later.

RISK FACTORS

- Frequent close or prolonged contact with an infected person
- Immunosuppression; poor nutrition; crowded living conditions
- Increasing age, ↑in ethnic minorities and foreign-born people

COMPLICATIONS

- Pleural effusion, pneumonia, other organ involvement

RECOGNIZE AND ANALYZE CUES

- Fatigue, malaise, anorexia, weight loss
- Chronic dry cough progressing to productive mucopurulent (often blood-streaked) cough
- Low-grade fever and night sweats
- Hemoptysis (advanced condition)
- May present with acute symptoms (fever, chills, flu-like symptoms, productive cough, pleuritic pain)
- Diagnostics: chest x-ray; sputum culture (three consecutive specimens); positive TB skin test means that the person has, at some time been, infected with the TB bacillus and developed antibodies; does not mean that the person has an active TB infection

MEDICAL MANAGEMENT: GENERATE SOLUTIONS

- Drugs: multiple antituberculosis medications

NURSING MANAGEMENT: TAKE ACTION

1. Initiate airborne respiratory isolation for the hospitalized patient (active TB).
2. Monitor respiratory status and improve effective airway clearance.
3. Promote diet with adequate protein; iron; vitamins A, B, C, and E; fresh produce. Avoid alcohol use.
4. Teach about importance of maintaining medication regimen and returning for sputum checks every 2 to 4 weeks.

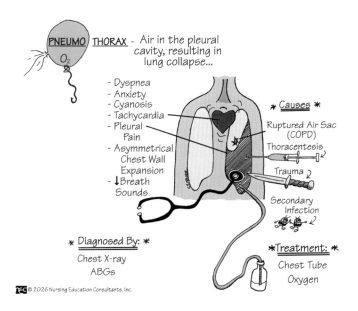

PNEUMO THORAX – Air in the pleural cavity, resulting in lung collapse...

- Dyspnea
- Anxiety
- Cyanosis
- Tachycardia
- Pleural Pain
- Asymmetrical Chest Wall Expansion
- ↓Breath Sounds

* Causes *

Ruptured Air Sac (COPD)

Thoracentesis

Trauma

Secondary Infection

* Diagnosed By: *

Chest X-ray
ABGs

*Treatment: *

Chest Tube
Oxygen

What You Need to Know
Pneumothorax

DEFINITION

Pneumothorax is air in the pleural space causing a loss of negative pressure, leading to the collapse or atelectasis of that portion of the lung. Types of pneumothorax include spontaneous pneumothorax (rupture of small blebs), tension pneumothorax (air enters pleural space and cannot escape), and hemothorax (collection of blood in pleural space).

RISK FACTORS

- Ruptured bleb (spontaneous)
- Thoracentesis
- Infection
- Trauma (penetrating or blunt chest injury)

COMPLICATIONS

- Respiratory failure, heart failure, death

RECOGNIZE AND ANALYZE CUES

- Diminished or absent breath sounds on the affected side
- Dyspnea, hypoxia, tachycardia, tachypnea
- Sudden onset of persistent chest pain, pain on the affected side when breathing
- Asymmetric chest wall expansion
- Hyperresonance on percussion of the affected side
- Possible development of a tension pneumothorax→ death
  - Severe dyspnea, marked tachycardia, profuse diaphoresis
  - Tracheal shift from the midline toward the unaffected side (late sign)

MEDICAL MANAGEMENT: GENERATE SOLUTIONS

- Insertion of a chest tube and O_2 therapy

NURSING MANAGEMENT: TAKE ACTION

1. Prehospital care: cover wound with occlusive dressing (secured on three sides so dressing has a vent).
2. Place in a semi-Fowler position and initiate O_2 therapy.
3. Establish and maintain water-sealed chest drainage system.
4. Have the patient cough and deep breathe every 2 hours.

ACUTE RESPIRATORY DISTRESS SYNDROME
(ARDS)

My heart is racing and I can't catch my breath

WHITE LUNG

VENT-O-MATIC

Signs & Symptoms
Tachypnea
Dyspnea
Retractions
Hypoxia
Tachycardia
↓Pulmonary Compliance

ABGs
↓Po_2 ↑Dyspnea
(Refractory Hypoxia - no improvement in O_2 sats with ↑FiO_2)

Causes
* Trauma
* Pulmonary Infection/ Aspiration
* Prolonged Ventilator Assistance
* MODS, SIRS
* Shock
* Fat Emboli
* Sepsis

What You Need to Know
Acute Respiratory Distress Syndrome

DEFINITION

Acute respiratory distress syndrome or noncardiogenic pulmonary edema, also re-ferred to as shock lung and white lung, is a condition characterized by increased capillary permeability in the alveolar capillary membrane, resulting in fluid leaking into the interstitial spaces and the alveoli and a decrease in pulmonary compliance.

RISK FACTORS

- Sepsis (most common)

COMPLICATIONS

- Multiple organ dysfunction syndrome (MODS) → Death

RECOGNIZE AND ANALYZE CUES

- Restlessness, confusion, tachypnea, dyspnea → profound respiratory distress
- Refractory hypoxemia (increasing hypoxia not responding to increased levels of fraction of inspired O_2 [FiO_2])
- Diagnostics: chest x-ray, ABGs, CT scan

MEDICAL MANAGEMENT: GENERATE SOLUTIONS

- Endotracheal intubation and mechanical ventilation
  - Positive end-expiratory pressure (PEEP)
  - Continuous positive airway pressure (CPAP)
- Alternative ventilation strategies
  - Airway pressure-release ventilation (APRV)
  - High-frequency oscillatory (HFO) ventilation
- Hemodynamic pressure monitoring

NURSING MANAGEMENT: TAKE ACTION

1. Maintain airway patency and improve ventilation.
2. Anticipate intubation or tracheotomy.
3. Endotracheal tube or tracheotomy suctioning.
4. Evaluate ABG reports, monitor hemoglobin and hematocrit, and SpO_2.
5. Sedation and paralytic agents are required to tolerate alternative modes of ventilation.
6. Positioning (prone to assist with redistribution of blood flow to less damaged areas of the lungs).

Important nursing interventions	Serious/life-threatening implications
Common signs & symptoms	Patient teaching

OBSTRUCTIVE SLEEP APNEA

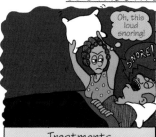

Symptoms

- Loud Snoring
- Excessive day time sleepiness
- Frequent episodes of obstructed breathing during sleep
- Morning headache
- Unrefreshing sleep
- Increased irritability

Treatments

Nonsurgical
- Change sleep position
- Decrease weight
- CPAP (Continuous Positive Airway Pressure)
- Drug Therapy for Underlying Cause

Surgical
- Adenoidectomy
- Uvulectomy
- Remodeling posterior oropharynx
- Bariatric surgery to ↓weight

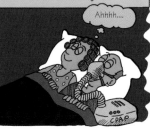

© 2026 Nursing Education Consultants, Inc.

What You Need to Know
Obstructive Sleep Apnea

DEFINITION

Obstructive sleep apnea is a disorder in which an individual frequently stops breathing during sleep (cessation of breathing for 10 seconds or longer occurring at least five times per hour). The individual may not be aware of snoring or apneic episodes. Apneic episodes cause recurrent arousals from sleep.

RISK FACTORS

- Obstruction by the soft palate or tongue; obesity

COMPLICATIONS

- Hypertension, stoke, dysrhythmias, type 2 diabetes

RECOGNIZE AND ANALYZE CUES

- Cardinal symptoms: 3 S's—snoring, sleepiness, and significant-other report of sleep apnea episodes
- Sleeper awakens after 10 seconds or longer of apnea
- Disruptive snoring, unrefreshing sleep, gasping while sleeping
- Short-term memory loss, morning headaches
- Driving accidents (falling asleep)
- Increasing irritability, personality changes, and depression
- Diagnostics: overnight polysomnography—sleep study

MEDICAL MANAGEMENT: GENERATE SOLUTIONS

- CPAP during sleep
- Surgery: Uvulopalatopharyngoplasty (UPPP) to remove the tonsils and adenoids and resect the uvula, the posterior part of the soft palate, and any excessive pharyngeal tissue.

NURSING MANAGEMENT: TAKE ACTION

1. Elevate the head of the bed and encourage to sleep on the side.
2. Encourage weight loss program if overweight.
3. Reinforce teaching about the proper use of equipment.
4. Teach about the dangers of driving or using heavy equipment due to daytime sleepiness.

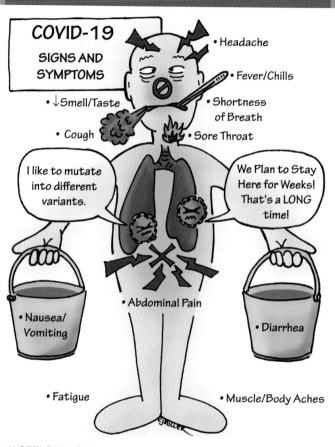

What You Need to Know
COVID-19 Signs and Symptoms

DEFINITION

Coronavirus disease (COVID-19) is an infectious respiratory disease caused by the SARS-CoV-2 virus and is responsible for the 2020 pandemic.

RISK FACTORS

- Older adults, immunosuppressed
- Underlying heart, lung, or diabetes conditions

COMPLICATIONS

- Acute respiratory failure, long COVID-19

RECOGNIZE AND ANALYZE CUES

- Fever or chills, cough
- Shortness of breath or difficulty breathing
- Fatigue, muscle, or body aches
- Headache, new loss of taste or smell
- Sore throat, congestion, or runny nose
- Nausea, vomiting, diarrhea
- Children have fewer symptoms than adults
- Asymptomatic
- Unique features: conjunctivitis, venous thromboembolic disease, encephalopathy with agitated delirium, reddish nodules on distal digits (in young adults)
- Diagnostics: viral testing (nasal or oral swabs; saliva)

MEDICAL MANAGEMENT: GENERATE SOLUTIONS

- O_2 in high concentration; intubation and mechanical ventilation
  - Use of BiPAP
  - Sedation (morphine) or muscle-paralyzing agents to allow controlled ventilation
- Drugs: antiviral medication (remdesivir), immune modulators (baricitinib, tocilizumab), convalescent plasma (recovered patients donate plasma and their antibodies are used in treatment)
- Preventative: COVID-19 vaccination and booster(s)

NURSING MANAGEMENT: TAKE ACTION

1. Monitor for difficulty breathing, persistent pain or pressure in the chest, new onset of confusion, cyanosis; may rapidly deteriorate 1 week after the onset of illness.
2. N95 respirator mask with a face shield for HCPs.
3. Teach prevention measures.
   - Wear a facemask; cough in the elbow area of arm; hands away from the eyes, nose, and mouth.
   - Avoid close contact; keep a distance of at least 6 feet.
   - Clean and disinfect frequently touched surfaces daily; wash hands frequently.

PROGRESSION OF ATHEROSCLEROSIS

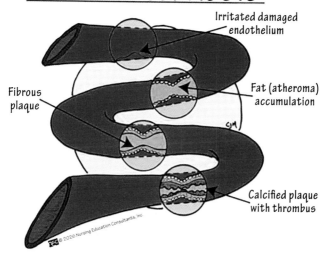

Irritated damaged endothelium

Fat (atheroma) accumulation

Fibrous plaque

Calcified plaque with thrombus

What You Need to Know

Progression of Atherosclerosis

DEFINITION

Atherosclerosis is a gradual thickening and narrowing of the arterial lumen; sometimes referred to as "hardening of the arteries." The process can occur in any artery of the body.

MODIFIABLE RISK FACTORS

- Total cholesterol level: >200 mg/dL
- High-density lipoprotein (HDL) ("good" cholesterol) levels: females <50 mg/dL; males <40 mg/dL
- Low-density lipoprotein (LDL) ("bad" cholesterol) levels: >130 mg/dL
- Triglyceride levels: ≥150 mg/dL
- Sedentary lifestyle, obesity, metabolic syndrome, stress, smoking

NONMODIFIABLE RISK FACTORS

- Genetic predisposition, family history, increasing age
- Ethnicity, sex (males ↑risk than females until age 55)

RECOGNIZE AND ANALYZE CUES

- Arteries commonly affected by atherosclerosis and the ensuing problems:
  - Coronary arteries: myocardial infarction
  - Cerebrovascular arteries: stroke, brain attack
  - Aorta: aortic aneurysm, peripheral vascular disease
  - Renal arteries: hypertension, kidney failure
  - Peripheral arteries: peripheral vascular disease

MEDICAL MANAGEMENT: GENERATE SOLUTIONS

- Decrease risk factors (exercise, stop smoking, ↓weight, ↓stress, ↓decrease fat in diet)
- Drugs: antihyperlipidemic and peripheral vasodilating medications

NURSING MANAGEMENT: TAKE ACTION

1. Identify patients at high risk.
   - Teach strategies on how to reduce modifiable risk factors.
   - Recognize significant deviations from laboratory values.
2. Reduce total fat and saturated fat intake.
3. Take prescribed drugs for lipid reduction.
4. Adjust total caloric intake to achieve and maintain ideal body weight.
5. Engage in daily physical activity (5 days/wk for 30 minutes).
6. Increase amount of complex carbohydrates, fiber, and vegetable proteins in diet.
7. Begin a tobacco cessation program.

HYPERTENSION

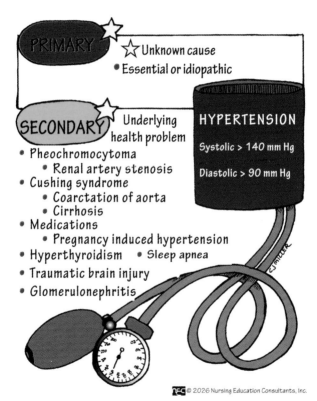

PRIMARY

Unknown cause
- Essential or idiopathic

SECONDARY Underlying health problem

HYPERTENSION

Systolic > 140 mm Hg

Diastolic > 90 mm Hg

- Pheochromocytoma
  - Renal artery stenosis
- Cushing syndrome
  - Coarctation of aorta
  - Cirrhosis
- Medications
  - Pregnancy induced hypertension
- Hyperthyroidism • Sleep apnea
- Traumatic brain injury
- Glomerulonephritis

— What You Need to Know —

Hypertension

DEFINITION

Hypertension or high blood pressure (BP) is an elevation above the normal limit, which is defined by the Joint National Committee 8 and the International Society of Hypertension as:

- Age <60 years: systolic BP (SBP) ≥140 mm Hg and/or diastolic BP (DBP) ≥90 mm Hg at two or more visits
- Age ≥60 years: SBP ≥150 mm Hg and/or DBP ≥90 mm Hg at two or more visits
- With diabetes or chronic kidney disease: SBP ≥140 mm Hg and/or DBP ≥90 mm Hg

RISK FACTORS

- Family history, obesity, alcohol use, excess dietary sodium
- Stress, physical inactivity, tobacco use, insulin resistance, obstructive sleep apnea

COMPLICATIONS

- Hypertensive heart disease, cerebrovascular disease
- Peripheral vascular disease nephrosclerosis, eyes (retinal damage)

RECOGNIZE AND ANALYZE CUES

- Known as the "silent killer" because it is often asymptomatic
- Headaches, facial flushing (redness), dizziness, or fainting
- Fatigue, palpitations, angina, dyspnea

MEDICAL MANAGEMENT: GENERATE SOLUTIONS

- Lifestyle modifications
    - Weight loss
    - Plant-based and Mediterranean diet with ↑fruit, nut, vegetable, legumes, and lean proteins—fish
    - Sodium restriction
    - Moderate-to-minimum alcohol use
    - Regular exercise program
    - Smoking cessation
- Drugs: antihypertensive agents
    - Adrenergic inhibitors
    - Angiotensin-converting enzyme (ACE) inhibitors
    - Angiotensin II receptor blockers (ARBs)
    - Calcium channel blockers (CCBs)
    - Direct vasodilators
- Diuretics
- *First-line drug classes are a thiazide diuretic (usually ordered first), a CCB, an ACE inhibitor or ARB.*

HYPERTENSION NURSING CARE

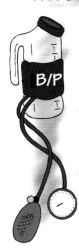

Daily weight

I & O

Urine output

Response of BP

Electrolytes

Take pulses

Ischemic episodes (TIA)

Complications: 4 Cs

    CAD

    CKD

    CHF

    CVA

© 2026 Nursing Education Consultants, Inc.

What You Need to Know
Hypertension Nursing Care

DEFINITION

Nursing management goals for the patient include the following:
- Achieve and maintain the goal of a lower BP
- Have minimal medication side effects
- Promote lifestyle modifications

NURSING MANAGEMENT: TAKE ACTION

1. Identify and educate high-risk individuals.
   - Decrease weight; regular BP checkups.
   - Avoid all tobacco products; limit alcohol and caffeine intake.
   - Control diabetes; engage in regular exercise.
   - Teach to take and record BP daily, including any symptoms.
2. Educate patient and family members on how to take BP.
   - Should be seated with arm at heart level.
   - No tobacco products or caffeine 30 minutes before taking BP.
   - Use appropriate cuff size; do not cross legs.
   - Use either upper arm or forearm for accurate readings.
3. Assess response to medication regimen.
   - Plan a method to keep track of medications (e.g., using daily pill box or marking on calendar).
   - Instruct about possible side effects, especially first-dose effect (orthostatic hypotension).
   - Teach to not suddenly stop taking medications; report side effects to healthcare provider.
     - Assure that side effects are often temporary.
     - Sexual problems (i.e., impotence) should be reported.
4. Teach about nutrition.
   - Encourage the Dietary Approaches to Stop Hypertension (DASH) eating plan (i.e., several servings of fish each week, plenty of fruits and vegetables, increasing fiber intake, increasing fluids [water]).
   - Review foods for a low-sodium and low-cholesterol diet.

Important nursing interventions	Serious/life-threatening implications
Common signs & symptoms	Patient teaching

HYPERTENSIVE CRISIS

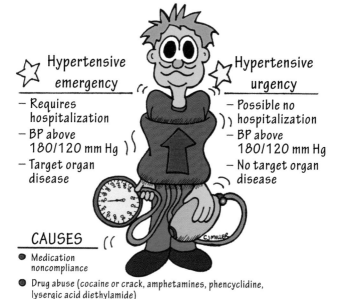

☆ Hypertensive emergency

- Requires hospitalization
- BP above 180/120 mm Hg
- Target organ disease

☆ Hypertensive urgency

- Possible no hospitalization
- BP above 180/120 mm Hg
- No target organ disease

CAUSES

● Medication noncompliance

● Drug abuse (cocaine or crack, amphetamines, phencyclidine, lysergic acid diethylamide)

● Head injury

● Preeclampsia/Eclampsia

● Pheochromocytoma

● MAOI meds with tyramine-containing foods

● Acute aortic dissection

What You Need to Know
Hypertensive Crisis

DEFINITION

Hypertensive crisis is defined as a systolic BP $\geq$180 mm Hg and diastolic BP of $\geq$120 mm Hg and is either a hypertensive urgency or emergency. Hypertensive emergencies have evidence of target organ disease.

RISK FACTORS

- Non-adherence to medication regimen
- Undermedicated for hypertension treatment
- Drug use (cocaine, amphetamine)
- Head injury, pheochromocytoma, preeclampsia, eclampsia
- Taking a monoamine oxidase inhibitor with tyramine-containing foods

COMPLICATIONS

- Hypertensive emergency: encephalopathy, intracranial or subarachnoid hemorrhage, heart failure (HF), myocardial infarction (MI), kidney failure, dissecting aortic aneurysm, retinopathy
- Hypertensive urgency: chronic, stable complications such as stable angina, chronic HF, or prior MI or cerebrovascular accident (no threat of an acute event)

RECOGNIZE AND ANALYZE CUES

- Sudden ↑BP with severe headache, epistaxis
- Nausea, vomiting, seizures, confusion, coma

MEDICAL MANAGEMENT: GENERATE SOLUTIONS

- Admitted to ICU
- Drugs: IV antihypertensive medications—vasodilators (nitroprusside, nicardipine), adrenergic inhibitor (labetalol), nitroglycerin

NURSING MANAGEMENT: TAKE ACTION

1. Place in semi-Fowler position.
2. Administer O_2, monitor SpO_2 and VS.
3. Administer IV antihypertensive medications.
4. Monitor BP every 5 to 15 minutes until the diastolic pressure is below 90; avoid rapid lowering of BP.
5. Monitor for neurologic or cardiovascular complications—seizures, numbness, weakness, or tingling of extremities; dysrhythmias, chest pain.

PERIPHERAL VASCULAR DISEASE
ARTERIAL vs. VENOUS ULCERS

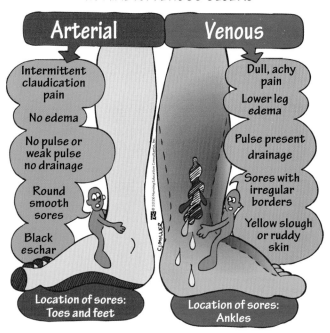

Arterial
- Intermittent claudication pain
- No edema
- No pulse or weak pulse no drainage
- Round smooth sores
- Black eschar
- Location of sores: Toes and feet

Venous
- Dull, achy pain
- Lower leg edema
- Pulse present drainage
- Sores with irregular borders
- Yellow slough or ruddy skin
- Location of sores: Ankles

=== **What You Need to Know** ===

Peripheral Vascular Disease

DEFINITION

Peripheral vascular disease is most commonly known as peripheral arterial disease (PAD); however, there is also peripheral venous disease. PAD involves narrowing and obstruction of the arteries, especially the lower extremities. Chronic arterial obstruction progressively leads to decreased oxygen delivery to the tissues. Peripheral venous disease or chronic venous insufficiency (CVI) is an alteration of the natural flow of blood through the veins of the peripheral circulation and is caused by thrombus formation (can lead to venous thromboembolism [VTE]) and/or defective valves. CVI leads to regurgitation of blood, venous pooling, and edema in the lower extremities, eventually resulting in the development of venous leg ulcers.

RISK FACTORS

- PAD: atherosclerosis, tobacco use, diabetes, hypertension, high cholesterol, age >60 years
- Venous thrombosis: immobility, age, obesity, major surgery, multiple traumas

COMPLICATIONS

- PAD: delayed healing, infection, necrosis, ulcerations, gangrene, amputation
- CVI: ulcerations, infection
- VTE: pulmonary embolism

RECOGNIZE AND ANALYZE CUES

- Review figure

MEDICAL MANAGEMENT: GENERATE SOLUTIONS

- PAD: ACE inhibitors, antiplatelet agents, clopidogrel, antihyperlipidemic, anticoagulant, antiplatelet, intermittent claudication (cilostazol, pentoxifylline), exercise (walking)
    - Surgery: percutaneous transluminal balloon angioplasty with stenting or atherectomy, peripheral arterial bypass graft
- CVI: graduated compression stockings, elevation of leg, oral and topical nonsteroidal antiinflammatory drugs, exercise (walking)
- VTE: anticoagulation therapy, pain relief, graduated compression stockings

NURSING MANAGEMENT: TAKE ACTION

1. PAD: alleviation of poor tissue perfusion and pain.
2. CVI: decrease edema and promote venous return.
3. Venous thrombosis: prevention of VTE.

Important nursing interventions	Serious/life-threatening implications
Common signs & symptoms	Patient teaching

VENOUS THROMBOEMBOLISM RISK FACTORS

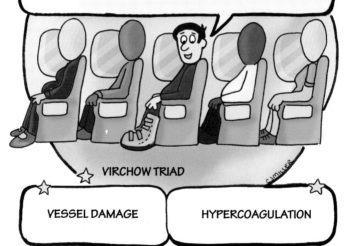

What You Need to Know
Venous Thromboembolism

DEFINITION

Venous thromboembolism (VTE) is the presence of a clot in a vein, which may be superficial (SVT) or a deep vein thrombosis (DVT). Phlebitis is inflammation of a superficial vein without the presence of a clot (thrombus).

RISK FACTORS (VIRCHOW TRIAD)

- *Venous stasis*: surgery (especially hip, pelvic, and orthopedic surgery), pregnancy, obesity, prolonged immobility, heart disease (atrial fibrillation, heart failure)
- *Hypercoagulability*: malignancies, dehydration, blood dyscrasias, oral contraceptives, hormone replacement therapy, pregnancy and postpartum
- *Endothelial damage*: IV fluids and drugs (IV catheterization, drug abuse, caustic solutions, or drugs), fractures and dislocations (especially of the pelvis, hip, or leg), history of VTE or diabetes

COMPLICATIONS

- Pulmonary embolus

RECOGNIZE AND ANALYZE CUES

- SVT: Firm, palpable, cordlike vein; area around vein is tender to touch, reddened, and warm; mild temperature elevation
- DVT: unilateral leg edema, pain, warm and tender to palpation, reddened, feeling of fullness in thigh or calf, ↑temperature (>100.4°F [38.0°C])

MEDICAL MANAGEMENT: GENERATE SOLUTIONS

- Drugs: anticoagulants, thrombolytics
- Surgery: Venous thrombectomy, vena cava interruption device

NURSING MANAGEMENT: TAKE ACTION

1. Initiate nursing measures to decrease venous stasis.
2. Anticipate rest and limb elevation with acute VTE, the ambulation.
3. Administer anticoagulation therapy.
   - Monitor for bleeding.
   - Evaluate laboratory tests for therapeutic range.
4. Monitor intermittent compression devices for high-risk patients.
5. Teach about the side effects of anticoagulants and the need for routine testing.

Important nursing interventions	Serious/life-threatening implications
Common signs & symptoms	Patient teaching

AORTIC DISSECTION

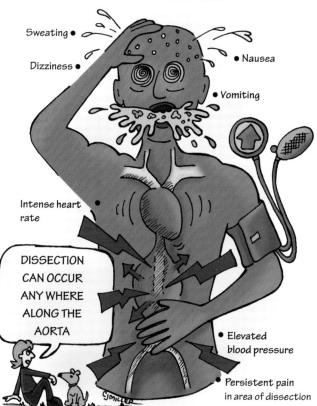

Aortic Dissection

DEFINITION

Aortic dissection, previously called *"dissecting aneurysm,"* is thought to be caused by a sudden tear in the aortic intima, allowing blood to enter the aortic wall. It is life threatening.

RISK FACTORS

- Chronic hypertension, genetic predisposition
- Male sex, nicotine use

COMPLICATIONS

- Cardiac tamponade

RECOGNIZE AND ANALYZE CUES

- Pain—"sharp," "tearing," "ripping," or "stabbing"
  - Depending on site of dissection— pain can be felt in the abdominal, back, neck, or anterior chest area
- Diaphoresis, nausea, vomiting
- Faintness, pallor, a rapid and weak pulse, apprehension
- Diagnosis: transesophageal echocardiography, computed tomographic angiography

MEDICAL MANAGEMENT: GENERATE SOLUTIONS

- Drugs: antihypertensives (goal of BP <120/80 mm Hg), morphine
- Surgery: endovascular stent graft

NURSING MANAGEMENT: TAKE ACTION

1. Administer medications (antihypertensives, morphine for pain).
2. Prepare for emergency surgery.
   - Evaluate characteristics of pulses in the lower extremities and mark them for evaluation and comparison after surgery.
   - Do not vigorously palpate the abdomen.
3. Provide postoperative care.
   - Monitor for hemorrhage, increasing abdominal girth, back pain, hypovolemia, and shock.
   - Check peripheral circulation, sensation, and movement hourly for the first 24 hours.
   - Monitor for graft occlusion—changes or ↓in quality of pulse, extremity cool below level of graft, change in color of extremity.
4. Teach the importance of keeping BP at the target level by taking antihypertensive medication.

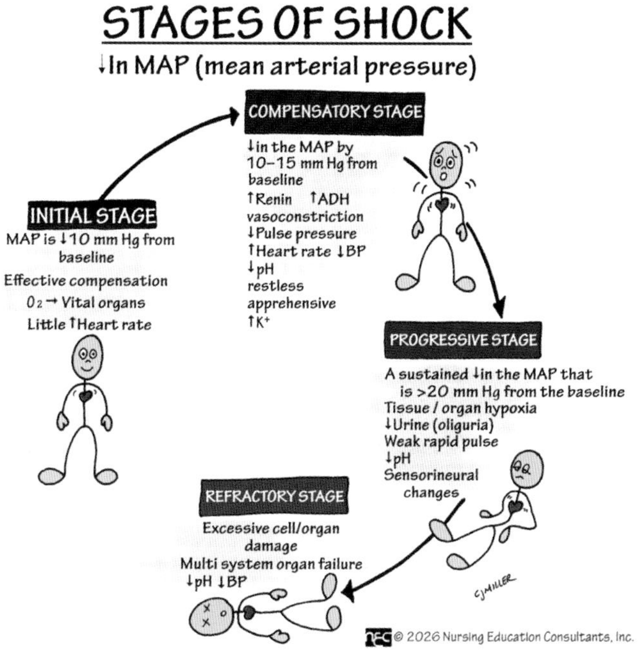

STAGES OF SHOCK
↓In MAP (mean arterial pressure)
INITIAL STAGE
MAP is ↓10 mm Hg from baseline
Effective compensation
O_2 → Vital organs
Little ↑Heart rate
COMPENSATORY STAGE
↓in the MAP by 10–15 mm Hg from baseline
↑Renin ↑ADH
vasoconstriction
↓Pulse pressure
↑Heart rate ↓BP
↓pH
restless
apprehensive
↑K^+
PROGRESSIVE STAGE
A sustained ↓in the MAP that is >20 mm Hg from the baseline
Tissue / organ hypoxia
↓Urine (oliguria)
Weak rapid pulse
↓pH
Sensorineural changes
REFRACTORY STAGE
Excessive cell/organ damage
Multi system organ failure
↓pH ↓BP
CJMILLER
© 2026 Nursing Education Consultants, Inc.

What You Need to Know
Stages of Shock

DEFINITION

Shock is a syndrome characterized by decreased tissue perfusion, impaired gas exchange, and cellular metabolism, which is life threatening. There are four main categories of shock—cardiogenic, hypovolemic, distributive (septic shock, neurogenic shock, anaphylactic), and obstructive (cardiac tamponade, tension pneumothorax, superior vena cava syndrome).

RECOGNIZE AND ANALYZE CUES

- Cardiogenic—heart pump failure
- Hypovolemic—loss of whole blood or body fluids
- Distributive
  - Septic shock—is a subset of sepsis with ↑mortality due to infection typically caused by bacteria
  - Neurogenic shock—occurs with spinal cord injury (within the first 30 minutes)
  - Anaphylactic—acute hypersensitivity and reaction to a sensitizing substance (drugs, chemicals, vaccine, food, insect venom)
- Obstructive—physical obstruction that causes heart to pump ineffectively

MEDICAL MANAGEMENT: GENERATE SOLUTIONS

- Treat underlying cause *first*
- Drugs to restore cardiac and other bodily functions depend on the type of shock

NURSING MANAGEMENT: TAKE ACTION

1. Identify patients at risk for developing shock.
2. Initiate O_2 therapy, treat pain, and alleviate anxiety.
3. Provide nursing interventions and medications to control or eliminate the cause.
4. Provide multisystem supportive care in intensive care setting.

Important nursing interventions	Serious/life-threatening implications
Common signs & symptoms	Patient teaching

CHRONIC STABLE ANGINA

OH, MY CHEST HURTS !!

CHARACTERISTICS

- Lasts <5 minutes
- Has the same cause each time
- Happens regularly
- Responds to nitroglycerin and rest

TRIGGERS

- Occurs usually during physical exertion or emotional stress
- Exposure to very hot or very cold temperatures
- After heavy meals
- Smoking

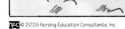

What You Need to Know
Chronic Stable Angina

DEFINITION

Chronic stable angina is chest discomfort or pain due to myocardial ischemia that is predictable and reproducible at a certain level of exertion, stress, or emotional upset. It is relieved by resting (stopping the activity that precipitated the pain), calming down from an emotional situation, or using sublingual nitroglycerin (NTC).

RISK FACTORS

- Hypertension, ↓high-density lipoprotein (HDL), ↑low-density lipoprotein (LDL), smoking, diabetes, obesity
- Sedentary lifestyle, chronic inflammation, kidney disease

COMPLICATIONS

- Acute coronary syndrome, dysrhythmias, heart failure, cardiac arrest

RECOGNIZE AND ANALYZE CUES

- Substernal chest pain
  - May radiate to the jaw, neck, shoulders, and/or arms
  - Feeling of indigestion or a burning sensation in the epigastric area
  - Pain may be felt between the shoulder blades
- Sweating, anxiety, heart palpitations
- Atypical symptoms in females and older adults
  - Dyspnea, nausea, mid-epigastric discomfort, and/or fatigue

MEDICAL MANAGEMENT: GENERATE SOLUTIONS

- Drugs: NTG (sublingual), long-acting nitrates, angiotensin-converting enzyme (ACE) inhibitors, β-blockers, and calcium channel blockers
- Surgery (coronary revascularization with coronary artery bypass surgery [CABG]) for patients who do not respond to medical management

NURSING MANAGEMENT: TAKE ACTION

1. Provide pain relief (NTG, opioid analgesic).
2. Apply supplemental O_2 and continuous electrocardiogram (ECG) monitoring.
3. Assess vital signs and obtain a 12-lead ECG.
4. Teach how to reduce modifiable risk factors.
5. Teach how to identify and avoid factors that precipitate angina.
6. Teach about drug therapy and side effects.

Important nursing interventions	Serious/life-threatening implications
Common signs & symptoms	Patient teaching

- MYOCARDIAL INFARCTION (MI) -
- CORONARY OCCLUSION -
- HEART ATTACK -

- Pain:
    Sudden Onset
    Substernal
    Crushing
    Tightness
    Severe
    Unrelieved by Nitroglycerin
    May Radiate To: Back
                 Neck
                 Jaw/Tooth

- Dyspnea   Shoulder
- Syncope (↓BP)   Arm
- Nausea
- Vomiting
- Extreme Weakness
- Diaphoresis
- Denial is
  Common
- ↑Pulse
- Changes in ST Segment

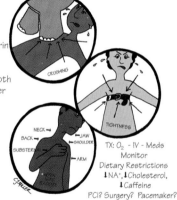

TX: O_2 - IV - Meds
    Monitor
Dietary Restrictions
  ↓NA⁺,↓Cholesterol,
    ↓Caffeine
PCI? Surgery? Pacemaker?

===== **What You Need to Know** =====
Myocardial Infarction

DEFINITION

Myocardial infarction (MI) occurs when myocardial tissue is abruptly and severely deprived of oxygen usually in a coronary artery by a thrombus caused by platelet aggregation. When blood flow to the heart is reduced by 80% to 90%, ischemia develops and causes irreversible myocardial cell death (necrosis) in the heart muscle beyond the blockage. There are two types of MI: non–ST-segment elevation myocardial infarction (NSTEMI) and ST-elevation myocardial infarction (STEMI).

RISK FACTORS

- Coronary artery disease (CAD)

COMPLICATIONS

- Dysrhythmias, heart failure (HF), cardiogenic shock, left ventricular aneurysm, acute pericarditis

RECOGNIZE AND ANALYZE CUES

- STEMI—an emergency situation caused by an occlusive thrombus with ST segment elevation
- NSTEMI—caused by a nonocclusive thrombus with ST segment depression and T wave inversion

MEDICAL MANAGEMENT: GENERATE SOLUTIONS

- STEMI—emergent percutaneous coronary intervention (PCI), thrombolytic therapy
- Antiplatelet therapy (e.g., chewable aspirin for unstable angina plus ticagrelor for STEMI and NSTEMI patients), IV nitroglycerin (NTG), and high-dose atorvastatin
- NSTEMI—systemic anticoagulation with either subcutaneous low-molecular-weight heparin (LMWH) or IV unfractionated heparin
- STEMI or NSTEMI—morphine, β-blockers, ACE inhibitors, angiotensin receptor blockers (ARBs)

NURSING MANAGEMENT: TAKE ACTION

1. Monitor vital signs, SpO_2 frequently; initiate continuous ECG monitoring.
   - Identify and treat life-threatening dysrhythmias quickly.
   - Assess for HF.
2. Promote rest and comfort; alleviate pain and reduce anxiety.
3. Teach about cardiac rehabilitation, physical activity, sexual activity, and drug therapy.

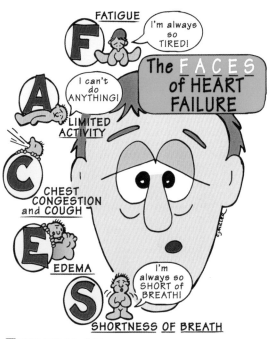

© 2026 Nursing Education Consultants, Inc.

What You Need to Know
FACES of Heart Failure

DEFINITION

Heart failure (HF), which is also called pump failure, is a common and chronic complex syndrome that is characterized by acute episodes requiring hospitalization. There are two types of HF—left-sided HF and right-sided HF. Acute decompensated heart failure (ADHF) is often a sudden increase in symptoms of HF with a decrease in functional status, often requiring immediate medical therapy and hospital admission. Chronic HF is a progressive and common syndrome where symptoms appear slowly over time and gradually worsen due to ↓cardiac output and ↑venous pressure associated with the death of heart muscle cells.

CLASSIFICATION AND STAGING HF

There are two different guidelines: the New York Heart Association (NYHA) functional system using numbers and the staging system developed by the American College of Cardiology and American Heart Association using letters.

A. Patients at high risk for developing HF (Class I NYHA)
B. Patients with cardiac structural abnormalities or remodeling who have not developed HF symptoms (Class I NYHA)
C. Patients with current or prior symptoms of HF (Class II or III NYHA)
D. Patients with refractory end-stage HF (Class IV NYHA)

RECOGNIZE AND ANALYZE CUES

- ADHF: pulmonary congestion (tachypnea, fatigue, pulmonary edema) and fluid volume overload (dyspnea, edema, weight gain)
- Chronic HF: fatigue, dyspnea, orthopnea, paroxysmal nocturnal dyspnea, nonproductive chronic cough, tachycardia, palpitations, edema, nocturia, sleep problems, weight changes
- Diagnostic: ↑B-type natriuretic peptide, urinalysis (proteinuria or microalbuminuria, ↑specific gravity)
  - Echocardiography, chest x-ray, ECG

Important nursing interventions   Serious/life-threatening implications

Common signs & symptoms   Patient teaching

LEFT-SIDED ♥ FAILURE

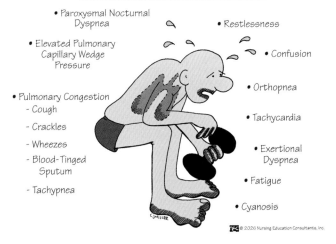

- Paroxysmal Nocturnal Dyspnea
- Elevated Pulmonary Capillary Wedge Pressure
- Pulmonary Congestion
  - Cough
  - Crackles
  - Wheezes
  - Blood-Tinged Sputum
  - Tachypnea

- Restlessness
- Confusion
- Orthopnea
- Tachycardia
- Exertional Dyspnea
- Fatigue
- Cyanosis

© 2026 Nursing Education Consultants, Inc.

=========== **What You Need to Know** ===========
Left-Sided Heart Failure

DEFINITION

Left-sided heart failure (HF) is the most common form of HF and begins with failure of the left ventricle and progresses to failure of both ventricles. Previously left-sided HF was called congestive heart failure (CHF); however, not all cases of left-sided ventricular failure involve fluid accumulation. There are two types of left-sided HF—systolic HF (HF with reduced ejection fraction [HFrEF]) and diastolic HF (HF with preserved left ventricular function [HFpEF]).

RISK FACTORS

- Hypertension, CAD, valvular heart disease
- Congenital heart defects, hyperthyroidism, cardiomyopathy

COMPLICATIONS

- Pleural effusion, dysrhythmias, hepatomegaly, death

RECOGNIZE AND ANALYZE CUES

- Think left-sided → lung congestion

MEDICAL MANAGEMENT: GENERATE SOLUTIONS

- Drugs
  - Acute decompensated HF: diuretics, vasodilators, morphine, positive inotropes (β-agonists, e.g., dopamine, dobutamine, norepinephrine, phosphodiesterase inhibitors [milrinone], digitalis).
  - Chronic HF: ACE inhibitors, ARBs, angiotensin neprilysin-angiotensin receptor (ARNI) inhibitor, aldosterone antagonist (spironolactone), β-adrenergic blockers
- Device therapy: cardiac resynchronization therapy (CRT) with biventricular pacing and internal cardioverter-defibrillator (ICD)

NURSING MANAGEMENT: TAKE ACTION

1. Provide nursing care during acute decompensated HF episode to manage problems of decreased cardiac output, impaired oxygenation, fluid overload, intolerance of physical activity, and managing a complex medication regimen.
2. Teach about self-management (medications, regular activity and rest, monitoring daily weight, diet [low sodium and limit fluids to 2 L/day], monitoring for worsening symptoms).

| Important nursing interventions | Serious/life-threatening implications |
| Common signs & symptoms | Patient teaching |

RIGHT-SIDED ♥ FAILURE
(Cor Pulmonale)

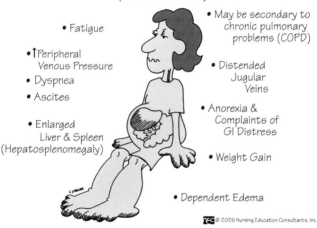

- Fatigue

- ↑Peripheral Venous Pressure
- Dyspnea
- Ascites

- Enlarged Liver & Spleen (Hepatosplenomegaly)

- May be secondary to chronic pulmonary problems (COPD)

- Distended Jugular Veins

- Anorexia & Complaints of GI Distress

- Weight Gain

- Dependent Edema

© 2026 Nursing Education Consultants, Inc.

===== **What You Need to Know** =====
Right-Sided Heart Failure

DEFINITION
Right-sided heart failure (HF) occurs when the right ventricle does not pump effectively. The most common cause of right-sided HF is left-sided HF. Cor pulmonale is right-sided HF caused by pulmonary disease (e.g., bronchitis, emphysema).

RISK FACTORS
- Left-sided HF
- Chronic pulmonary conditions, pulmonary embolus

COMPLICATIONS
- Life-threatening shortness of breath, extreme edema (ascites, anasarca)
- Shock, death

RECOGNIZE AND ANALYZE CUES
- Systemic congestion

MEDICAL MANAGEMENT: GENERATE SOLUTIONS
- Drugs—*treat underlying pulmonary disease*
  - Acute decompensated HF: diuretics, vasodilators, morphine, positive inotropes (β-agonists, e.g., dopamine, dobutamine, norepinephrine, phosphodiesterase inhibitors [milrinone], digitalis).
  - Chronic HF: ACE inhibitors, ARBs, ARNI inhibitor, aldosterone antagonist (spironolactone), β-adrenergic blockers
- Continuous, long-term O_2 therapy

NURSING MANAGEMENT: TAKE ACTION
1. Assess for dependent edema—ankles and legs; if on bedrest, fluid accumulates in the sacrum area.
2. Monitor daily weight—*remember weight is the most reliable indicator of fluid gain and loss*.
3. Teach about self-management (medications, regular activity and rest, monitoring daily weight, diet [low sodium and limit fluids to 2 L/day], monitoring for worsening symptoms).

Important nursing interventions	Serious/life-threatening implications
Common signs & symptoms	Patient teaching

TREATING HEART FAILURE

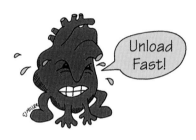

Unload Fast!

- **U**pright Position
- **N**itrates
- **L**asix
- **O**xygen
- **A**CE Inhibitors, ARBs
- **D**igoxin

- **F**luids (Decrease)
- **A**fterload (Decrease)
- **S**odium Restriction
- **T**est (Digoxin Level, ABGs, BNP, Potassium Level)

What You Need to Know
Treating Heart Failure

DEFINITION

The general management of HF is initially to treat the underlying cause, administer drugs, provide and care for device therapy (cardiac resynchronization therapy [CRT] with biventricular pacing and internal cardioverter-defibrillator [ICD]), monitor daily weight, maintain a low sodium and possible fluid-restricted diet, and initiate O_2 by mask or nasal cannula as needed. There are a variety of mnemonics to help you remember the various treatment regimens for HF.

BANDAID

Beta-blocker—metoprolol, cavedilol, bisoprolol
Angiotensin-converting enzyme inhibitor, ARB
Nitrate—hydralazine or potentially a neprilysin inhibitor
Diuretics—loop (furosemide), thiazide
Aldosterone antagonist—spironolactone
Ivabradine—selective sinoatrial node inhibitor
Devices—ICD, CRT, or both and digoxin

   Adapted from Chia, N., Fulcher, J., & Keech, A. (2015). Beta-blocker, angiotensin-converting enzyme inhibitor/angiotensin receptor blocker, nitrate-hydralazine, diuretics, aldosterone antagonist, ivabradine, devices and digoxin (BANDAID²): An evidence-based mnemonic for the treatment of systolic heart failure. *Internal Medicine Journal, 46*(6), 653-662. https://doi.org/10.1111/imj.12839

DAD BOND CLASH

D: Digitalis
A: ACE inhibitors
D: Dobutamine

B: Beta-blockers
O: Oxygen
N: Nitrates
D: Diuretics

C: Calcium channel blockers
L: Lifestyle changes
A: Angiotensin II receptor blockers
S: Sodium restriction
H: Hydralazine

   From Vera, M. (2023, July 12 updated). Management of heart failure: "DAD BOND CLASH." *Nurseslabs.* https://nurseslabs.com/cardiovascular-care-nursing-mnemonics-tips/

NORMAL ELIMINATION

PROMOTE ELIMINATION

P • Position - Upright, sitting
O • Output - Adequate hydration
O • Offer Fluids
P • Privacy
E • Exercise
R • Report Results

OBSERVE

S • Size (Amount)
C • Consistency
O • Occult Blood
O • Odor
P • Peristalsis

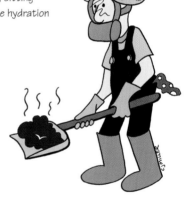

Gastrointestinal

What You Need to Know
Normal Elimination

DEFINITION

Normal elimination of bowel waste products is essential for body functioning. Elimination patterns and habits vary among patients and an alteration in elimination is often an early sign of a problem in the gastrointestinal (GI) tract or other body systems.

FACTORS INFLUENCING BOWEL ELIMINATION

- Age—age 2 to 3 control defecation; older adult may have difficulty controlling defecation
- Diet—fiber provides bulk for fecal material
- Fluid intake—fluid intake of 3.7 L/day males; 2.7 L/day females is recommended
- Physical activity—promotes peristalsis
- Psychological factors—stress ↑GI motility
- Personal habits—influence bowel function
- Position during defecation—squatting or sitting is normal position
- Pain—defecation should be painless
- Pregnancy—may have constipation and hemorrhoids
- Surgery and anesthesia—medications slow peristalsis
- Medications—some affect bowel function (laxatives)
- Diagnostic tests—often require a bowel prep

COMMON BOWEL ELIMINATION PROBLEMS

- Constipation—can be caused by improper diet, ↓fluid intake, lack of exercise, certain medications
- Impaction—unrelieved constipation → hardened feces
- Diarrhea—loose, liquid stools → dehydration, fluid/electrolyte loss
- Incontinence—inability to control feces and gas
- Flatulence—can cause abdominal fullness, pain, cramping
- Hemorrhoids—dilated, engorged veins lining the rectum; can be internal or external

---

Important nursing interventions	Serious/life-threatening implications
Common signs & symptoms	Patient teaching

APPENDICITIS

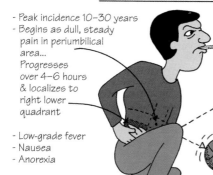

- Peak incidence 10–30 years
- Begins as dull, steady pain in periumbilical area... Progresses over 4–6 hours & localizes to right lower quadrant

- Low-grade fever
- Nausea
- Anorexia

- Sudden pain relief may indicate rupture of appendix (Leads to peritonitis)

Diagnosis
- Clinical signs and symptoms
- ↑WBC
- Abdominal Ultrasound, CT Scan

- Rebound Pain or Tenderness (RLQ) at McBurney's Point

*Treatment *
- Emergency Appendectomy
- IV Fluids & Antibiotics

C.J.MILLER

===== **What You Need to Know** =====

Appendicitis

DEFINITION

Appendicitis is the inflammation and obstruction of the appendix, leading to bacterial infection. If appendicitis is not treated, the appendix can become gangrenous and burst, causing peritonitis and septicemia, which could progress to death. It is the most common cause of acute abdominal pain.

RISK FACTORS

- Age: peak at 10 to 30 years of age
- Diet: diet low in fiber and high in refined sugars and carbohydrates.
- Obstruction to opening of appendix: hardened fecal matter, foreign bodies, or microorganisms

COMPLICATIONS

- Rupture of the appendix, abscess
- Peritonitis

RECOGNIZE AND ANALYZE CUES

- Colicky, cramping, abdominal pain located around the umbilicus then migrating toward McBurney's point (right lower quadrant); pain worsens with time
- Anorexia, low-grade fever, rebound tenderness
- Diagnostic: ↑white blood cell (WBC), abdominal ultrasound, CT scan

MEDICAL MANAGEMENT: GENERATE SOLUTIONS

- Surgery: appendectomy

NURSING MANAGEMENT: TAKE ACTION

1. Provide preoperative care.
   - Keep NPO, initiate an IV access, monitor VS.
   - Administer analgesics and antiemetics as ordered.
   - Allow a position of comfort.
2. Provide postoperative care.
   - Discharge usually within 24 hours if no complications.
   - Ambulation started a few hours after surgery.
   - Diet is advanced as tolerated.
   - If perforation occurs, patient is kept longer to receive IV antibiotics.

PERITONITIS

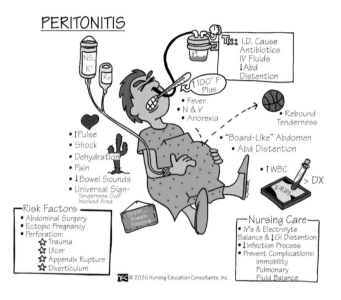

Tx: I.D. Cause
Antibiotics
IV Fluids
↓Abd Distention

NS, K⁺

Rx

100° F Plus
- Fever
- N & V
- Anorexia

- •Rebound Tenderness
- "Board-Like" Abdomen
- Abd Distention

- •↑Pulse
- Shock
- Dehydration
- Pain
- ↓Bowel Sounds
- Universal Sign-
Tenderness Over Involved Area

- •↑WBC

X-Ray > DX

SHHH... Bowels Sleeping

Risk Factors
- Abdominal Surgery
- Ectopic Pregnancy
- Perforation:
  - ☆ Trauma
  - ☆ Ulcer
  - ☆ Appendix Rupture
  - ☆ Diverticulum

Nursing Care
- IV's & Electrolyte Balance & ↓GI Distention
- ↓Infection Process
- Prevent Complications:
  Immobility
  Pulmonary
  Fluid Balance

© 2026 Nursing Education Consultants, Inc.

What You Need to Know
Peritonitis

DEFINITION

Peritonitis results from a localized or generalized inflammatory process of the peritoneum. It may occur when abdominal organs perforate or rupture and release their contents (bile, enzymes, hydrochloric acid, and bacteria) into the normal sterile peritoneal cavity. It is a life-threatening condition.

RISK FACTORS

- Ruptured appendix, ruptured ectopic pregnancy
- Abdominal penetrating trauma, peritoneal dialysis
- Perforation of an ulcer or diverticulum, intestinal cancer

COMPLICATIONS

- Septicemia, septic shock

RECOGNIZE AND ANALYZE CUES

- Sharp or knifelike pain and/or dull and deep-seated pain over involved area; rebound tenderness; pain may radiate to back, shoulder, or scapula
  - Sudden, excruciating pain suggests the possibility of rupture
- Abdominal muscle rigidity ("board-like" abdomen), guarding
- Tachycardia, hypotension, shallow respirations
- Diagnostics: ↑WBC, hemoconcentration from fluid shifts, abdominal x-ray, CT scan, ultrasonography

MEDICAL MANAGEMENT: GENERATE SOLUTIONS

- Drugs: opioid analgesics, antibiotics, antiemetics
- NG tube, NPO, IV fluid/electrolytes
- Surgery

NURSING MANAGEMENT: TAKE ACTION

1. Administer analgesics for pain.
2. Position in semi-Fowler to localize drainage and prevent the spread of infection.
3. Monitor for complications.

BOWEL OBSTRUCTION

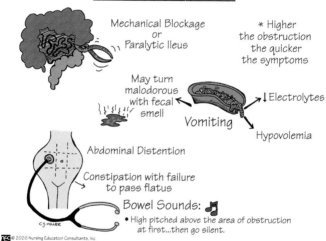

Mechanical Blockage
or
Paralytic Ileus

* Higher
the obstruction
the quicker
the symptoms

May turn
malodorous
with fecal
smell

↓ Electrolytes

Vomiting

Hypovolemia

Abdominal Distention

Constipation with failure
to pass flatus

Bowel Sounds: ♫
- High pitched above the area of obstruction
at first...then go silent.

C.J. MILLER

What You Need to Know
Bowel Obstruction

DEFINITION

A bowel obstruction, or intestinal obstruction, occurs when intestinal contents cannot pass through the GI tract due to interference with normal peristalsis and impairment of the forward flow of intestinal contents. It is a potentially life-threatening condition. Bowel obstructions are either mechanical or nonmechanical and may have partial or complete blockage.

RISK FACTORS

- Previous abdominal surgery, hernia
- Chronic constipation, cholelithiasis
- Inflammatory bowel disease, diverticular disease

COMPLICATIONS

- Infection/septicemia, gangrene, and/or perforation of the bowel
- Severe dehydration and electrolyte imbalances

RECOGNIZE AND ANALYZE CUES

- Colicky abdominal pain, nausea and vomiting, distention, constipation

MEDICAL MANAGEMENT: GENERATE SOLUTIONS

- Nasogastric suctioning and decompression
- Surgery, fluid/electrolyte replacement, antibiotics

NURSING MANAGEMENT: TAKE ACTION

1. Maintain NPO status and nasogastric (NG) suction.
2. Evaluate peristalsis, presence of any bowel function.
3. Assess for dehydration, hypovolemia, and electrolyte imbalance.
4. Monitor I&O including emesis and NG tube drainage.
5. Provide preoperative and postoperative care as indicated.
    - Postoperative: Monitor vital signs frequently and evaluate for the presence or escalation of infectious process, provide wound care, evaluate drainage and healing from abdominal drains and from abdominal incisional area.

TYPES OF BOWEL OBSTRUCTIONS

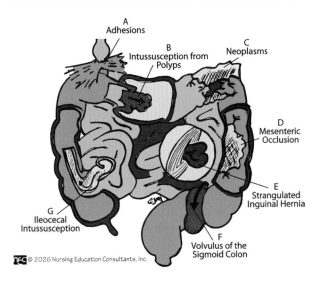

A
Adhesions

B
Intussusception from Polyps

C
Neoplasms

D
Mesenteric Occlusion

E
Strangulated Inguinal Hernia

F
Volvulus of the Sigmoid Colon

G
Ileocecal Intussusception

© 2026 Nursing Education Consultants, Inc.

===== **What You Need to Know** =====

Types of Bowel Obstructions

DEFINITION

Bowel obstructions or intestinal obstructions are either mechanical or nonmechanical and may have partial or complete blockage.

RISK FACTORS

- Surgical adhesions

COMPLICATIONS

- Septicemia, septic shock

TYPES OF OBSTRUCTIONS

- Mechanical
  - Strangulated hernia
  - Intussusception: the telescoping of one portion of the intestine into another (occurs most often in infants and small children)
  - Volvulus: twisting of the bowel
  - Tumors: cancer (most frequent cause of obstruction in older adults)
  - Adhesions (fibrous bands between tissues and organs after surgery)
  - Fecal impactions (especially in older adults)
  - Strictures due to Crohn's disease
  - Fibrosis due to endometriosis
- Nonmechanical
  - Paralytic ileus: lack of intestinal peristalsis and bowel sounds
  - Vascular obstructions: infarction of superior mesenteric artery

RECOGNIZE AND ANALYZE CUES

- Small intestine obstruction
  - Sudden onset of pain.
  - Vomiting—proximal obstruction: rapid development of nausea and vomiting that may be projectile and contain bile; distal obstruction: gradual onset of vomiting that is more fecal and foul smelling. *Remember ….bowel sounds may be high-pitched above the area of obstruction → silent or absent as paralytic ileus develops*.
- Large intestine obstruction
  - Abdominal distention, no flatus, persistent, cramping abdominal pain, vomiting rare. Bowel sounds present → become hypoactive.
- Both types—abdominal tenderness and rigidity, dehydration, sepsis, tachycardia, dry mucous membranes, hypotension, temperature >100°F (37.8°C).

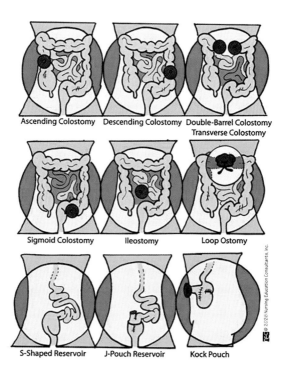

Ascending Colostomy   Descending Colostomy   Double-Barrel Colostomy
Transverse Colostomy

Sigmoid Colostomy   Ileostomy   Loop Ostomy

S-Shaped Reservoir   J-Pouch Reservoir   Kock Pouch

© 2026 Nursing Education Consultants, Inc.

What You Need to Know
Types of Ostomies

DEFINITION

A colostomy is a surgically created opening in the colon that allows the passage of stool, which is generally semisoft; bowel control may be achieved. The outermost part that is visible is called a stoma. An ileostomy is a surgically created opening in the ileum; stool drainage is liquid and excoriating; drainage is frequently continuous and difficult to establish bowel control. Kock pouch and Barnett Continent Intestinal Reservoir are two types of continent ileostomies.

NURSING MANAGEMENT: TAKE ACTION

1. Evaluate stoma after surgery; should remain pink and moist; dark blue stoma indicates ischemia.
2. Measure the stoma; select an appropriately sized appliance.
   - Anticipate mild-to-moderate swelling for the first 2 to 3 weeks after surgery, which necessitates changes in the size of the appliance.
   - Keep the skin around the stoma clean, dry, and free of stool and intestinal secretions.
   - Ostomy bags should be changed when they are about one-third full to avoid the weight of the bag dislodging the skin barrier.
3. Pouching an ostomy.
   - A pouching system consists of a pouch and a skin barrier (or wafer).
   - Pouches come in one- and two-piece systems and are flat or convex.
   - Pouches may have the opening precut by the manufacturer; others require the stoma opening to be cut by the nurse or patient to fit the stoma.
   - Pouch may have an integrated closure or may need a clip (older types).
   - Change the pouching system approximately every 2 to 4 days.

| Important nursing interventions | Serious/life-threatening implications |
| Common signs & symptoms | Patient teaching |

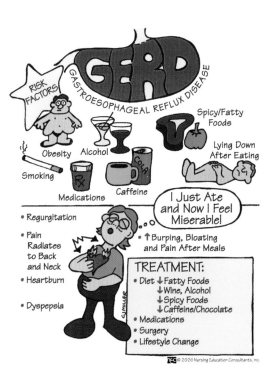

What You Need to Know
GERD

DEFINITION

Gastroesophageal reflux disease (GERD) is caused by the backward flow or reflux of gastric contents into the esophagus (esophageal reflux). The amount of damage depends on the amount and composition of gastric contents and the ability of the esophagus to remove the acidic fluids.

RISK FACTORS

- Incompetent lower esophageal sphincter
- Obesity, infection with *Helicobacter pylori*
- Alcohol, smoking, caffeine, spicy/fatty foods

COMPLICATIONS

- Esophagitis, Barrett esophagus (↑cancer risk)

RECOGNIZE AND ANALYZE CUES

- Dyspepsia (indigestion), regurgitation, pyrosis (heartburn)
- Feeling uncomfortably full, bloating, nausea, flatulence, belching, bloating
- Diagnostics: esophagogastroduodenoscopy

MEDICAL MANAGEMENT: GENERATE SOLUTIONS

- Drugs: proton pump inhibitors (PPIs), H_2-receptor blockers, antacids, prokinetics
- Endoscopic: intraluminal valvuloplasty, radiofrequency ablation
- Surgery: Nissen or Toupet fundoplication

NURSING MANAGEMENT: TAKE ACTION

1. Avoid drinking beverages during meals, including alcohol and carbonated drinks.
2. Do not eat or drink fluids 2 to 3 hours before bed or lie down for 1 to 2 hours after meals.
3. Eat four to six small meals per day (at 3-hour intervals); avoid foods that precipitate discomfort (fats, caffeine, chocolate, spicy food, tomato products).
4. Consume a high-protein, low-fat diet; avoid temperature extremes in foods.
5. If overweight, start a weight reduction program.
6. Elevate the head of the bed on 4- to 6-inch (10–15 cm) blocks or wedge-style pillow.

PEPTIC ULCER DISEASE

Gastric Ulcers
- Weight Loss
- Acid - Normal or Hyposecretion
- Pain ½ – 1 Hour After Meals
- Vomiting
- Eating may ↑ Pain

Common Risk Factors
- Stress
- H. pylori
- Alcohol
- Smoking
- Gastritis

Stress Ulcers
- Physiological Stress
- Shock
- Cushing's Ulcer - Brain Injury
- Curling's Ulcer- Extensive Burns Less Common

Duodenal Ulcers
- Most Common
- Well Nourished
- Pain 2–3 Hours After Meals
- Food May ↓ Pain

BUS STOP

What You Need to Know
Peptic Ulcer Disease

DEFINITION

Peptic ulcer disease (PUD) is an erosion of the GI mucosa by hydrochloric acid and pepsin. Any location in the GI tract that comes in contact with gastric secretions is susceptible to ulcer development. There are three types of ulcers: gastric, duodenal, and stress.

RISK FACTORS

- Infection with *Helicobacter pylori (H. pylori)*
- NSAID use
- ↑Alcohol intake, smoking

COMPLICATIONS

- GI bleeding, perforation, gastric outlet obstruction

RECOGNIZE AND ANALYZE CUES

- Review figure
- Diagnostics: endoscopy, serology test and biopsy for *H. pylori*, ↓hemoglobin and hematocrit

MEDICAL MANAGEMENT: GENERATE SOLUTIONS

- Drugs: antibiotics, bismuth (Pepto-Bismol), PPIs, H_2-receptor blockers, cytoprotective drugs, antacids
- Surgery: less common due to effective medication therapy

NURSING MANAGEMENT: TAKE ACTION

1. Promote measures to manage acute or persistent pain.
   - Administer medications; make modifications to diet.
2. Monitor for upper GI bleeding and other complications.
3. Teach about lifestyle modifications.
   - Eat a nonirritating or bland diet; although hot, rough, or spicy foods do not cause PUD, avoid them if they cause discomfort.
   - Minimize use of NSAIDs and anti-inflammatory medications.
   - Decrease or eliminate alcohol consumption and smoking.

CHRON'S DISEASE

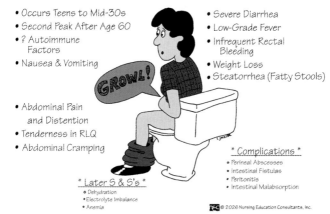

- Occurs Teens to Mid-30s
- Second Peak After Age 60
- ? Autoimmune Factors
- Nausea & Vomiting

- Abdominal Pain and Distention
- Tenderness in RLQ
- Abdominal Cramping

- Severe Diarrhea
- Low-Grade Fever
- Infrequent Rectal Bleeding
- Weight Loss
- Steatorrhea (Fatty Stools)

GROWL!

* Complications *
- Perineal Abscesses
- Intestinal Fistulas
- Peritonitis
- Intestinal Malabsorption

* Later S & S's *
- Dehydration
- Electrolyte Imbalance
- Anemia

© 2026 Nursing Education Consultants, Inc.

What You Need to Know
Crohn's Disease

DEFINITION

Crohn's disease (ileitis or enteritis) is inflammation occurring anywhere along the GI tract, from the mouth to the anus; patches of inflammation occur next to healthy bowel tissue; most frequently affects the distal ileum and proximal colon.

RISK FACTORS

- Cigarette smoking, diet ↑fat, refined sugars, processed foods

COMPLICATIONS

- Severe malabsorption, fistula, perforation

RECOGNIZE AND ANALYZE CUES

- Review figure

MEDICAL MANAGEMENT: GENERATE SOLUTIONS

- Drugs: anti-inflammatory: aminosalicylates (sulfasalazine), corticosteroids, immunomodulators (azathioprine, methotrexate), biologic and targeted medications (infliximab, adalimumab), antidiarrheals, probiotics
- Surgery indicated for bowel obstruction, hemorrhage, fistulas, perforation

NURSING MANAGEMENT: TAKE ACTION

1. Promote hemodynamic stability and hydration during the acute phase.
   - Evaluate adequate hydration status; monitor weight.
   - Encourage fluid intake of 2500 to 3000 mL/day.
   - Evaluate electrolyte status; monitor potassium level if on corticosteroids.
   - Assess characteristics and number of stools.
2. Promote adequate nutrition.
   - Balanced diet with increased protein and calories.
   - Assess for iron deficiency anemia.
   - Help identify and avoid foods that precipitate diarrhea.
   - Anticipate parenteral nutrition or enteral feeding.
3. Teach about exacerbations and remissions and ways to cope with stress and chronicity of condition.
4. Teach about medication regimen.

DUMPING SYNDROME

1 15

Occurs 15-30 Minutes
After Eating

- Weakness
  - Dizziness, Vertigo
    - Diaphoresis

- Tachycardia
- Abdominal Cramping
- Self-Limiting

- Epigastric
  Fullness

Stomach

High
Carbs
High
Fluids

- No Fluids
  With Meals
- No High Carbs
  i.e., Sweets,
  Milk

Duodenum

CJMILLER

What You Need to Know
Dumping Syndrome

DEFINITION

Dumping syndrome occurs when a large bolus of gastric chyme and hypertonic fluid enter the intestine in an abnormally fast manner. It is common after gastric or esophageal surgery.

RISK FACTORS

- Gastric or esophageal surgery
- Bariatric surgery

COMPLICATIONS

- Hypoglycemia
- Malnutrition, weight loss
- Electrolyte imbalance—hypokalemia

RECOGNIZE AND ANALYZE CUES

- Early symptoms—occurs within 15 to 30 minutes after eating
  - Vertigo, tachycardia, syncope, sweating, pallor, palpitations, desire to lie down
- Late symptoms—occurs 90 minutes to 3 hours after eating due to ↑insulin release
  - Dizziness, light-headedness, diaphoresis, confusion

MEDICAL MANAGEMENT: GENERATE SOLUTIONS

- Drugs: octreotide, acarbose

NURSING MANAGEMENT: TAKE ACTION

1. Teach measures to prevent dumping syndrome.
   - ↓amount of food eaten at one meal; eat small meals at 3-hour intervals.
   - ↓simple carbohydrates, ↑proteins, ↑fat.
   - Avoid milk and milk products.
   - No added fluids with meal; fluids between meals *only*.
   - ↓concentrated sweets (soda, candy, desserts).
   - Position in semirecumbent position during meals; may lie down on the left side for 20 to 30 minutes after meals to delay stomach emptying.
   - Hypoglycemia may occur 2 to 3 hours after eating, caused by the rapid entry of carbohydrates into jejunum.
2. Monitor for complications.

"SIR" HERNIA

Strangulated...

> Blood supply is
> cut off, emergency
> surgery situation.

Incarcerated...

> Hernia is trapped
> outside peritoneal
> cavity.

Reducible...

> Hernia moves
> back into
> peritoneal
> cavity.

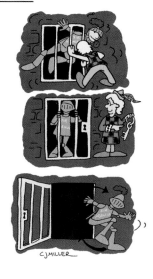

© 2026 Nursing Education Consultants, inc.

CJMILLER

What You Need to Know

SIR Hernia

DEFINITION

A hernia is a protrusion of the intestine through an abnormal opening or weakened area of the abdominal wall.

RISK FACTORS

- Chronic cough, obesity, pregnancy
- Straining during bowel movement or lifting heavy objects
- Males—more likely to have inguinal hernia
- Females—more likely to have femoral or umbilical hernia

COMPLICATIONS

- Incarceration, strangulation

RECOGNIZE AND ANALYZE CUES

- Pain, nausea, vomiting, bloating
- Visible as a protrusion through abdominal wall

MEDICAL MANAGEMENT: GENERATE SOLUTIONS

- Truss: pad that supports hernia
- Surgery: herniorrhaphy

NURSING MANAGEMENT: TAKE ACTION

1. Anticipate that any hernia that is not reducible needs immediate surgical evaluation.
2. Monitor for signs of strangulation—abdominal distention, nausea, vomiting, severe pain, fever, tachycardia.
3. Provide preoperative care—most often outpatient day surgery.
4. Provide postoperative care.
   - Assess males for development of scrotal edema; may require the use of a scrotal support with application of an ice bag.
   - Encourage deep breathing and activity.
   - If coughing occurs, teach how to splint the incision.
   - May need a stool softener to prevent constipation.
   - Refrain from heavy lifting (>10 lb) for approximately 6 to 8 weeks after surgery.
   - Keep the incision site clean and dry: use occlusive dressing or leave open to air.

CIRRHOSIS:
LATER CLINICAL MANIFESTATIONS

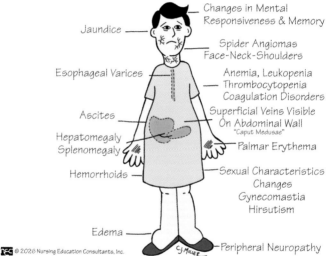

- Jaundice
- Changes in Mental Responsiveness & Memory
- Spider Angiomas Face-Neck-Shoulders
- Esophageal Varices
- Anemia, Leukopenia Thrombocytopenia Coagulation Disorders
- Ascites
- Superficial Veins Visible On Abdominal Wall "Caput Medusae"
- Hepatomegaly Splenomegaly
- Palmar Erythema
- Hemorrhoids
- Sexual Characteristics Changes Gynecomastia Hirsutism
- Edema
- Peripheral Neuropathy

CJ MILLER

===== **What You Need to Know** =====

Cirrhosis: Later Clinical Manifestations

DEFINITION

Hepatic cirrhosis is a chronic, progressive disease of the liver characterized by the degeneration and destruction of liver cells.

RISK FACTORS

- Chronic alcohol use, malnutrition, viral hepatitis
- Hepatitis nonalcoholic fatty liver disease, right-sided heart failure, obesity

COMPLICATIONS

- Portal hypertension, ascites, esophageal varices
- Biliary obstruction, hepatic encephalopathy (HE)

RECOGNIZE AND ANALYZE CUES

- Early symptoms—fatigue, enlarged liver, abnormal liver function tests
- Late symptoms—review figure

MEDICAL MANAGEMENT: GENERATE SOLUTIONS

- Conservative therapy: rest, B-complex vitamins, avoiding alcohol, aspirin, acetaminophen, NSAIDs
- Ascites: ↓sodium diet, diuretics, paracentesis
- Drugs (esophageal varices): β-blocker (e.g., propranolol), octreotide, vasopressin
- Drugs (HE): antibiotics (rifaximin), lactulose
- Esophageal varices: endoscopic band ligation or sclerotherapy, balloon tamponade, portacaval shunt, distal splenorenal shunt
- Transjugular intrahepatic portal-systemic shunt (TIPS)—nonsurgical procedure to relieve portal hypertension

NURSING MANAGEMENT: TAKE ACTION

1. Promote nutrition: ↑calories, carbohydrates, moderate to ↓fat levels, vitamin supplements.
2. Manage ascites: ↓sodium diet, diuretics, paracentesis.
3. Monitor for esophageal varices; hemorrhage.
   - Initiate rescue therapy with esophageal tamponade balloon.
   - Monitor for spontaneous bacterial peritonitis following variceal hemorrhage.
4. Assess and manage HE: ↓ammonia formation.
5. Teach to avoid acetaminophen, alcohol, smoking; diet; measures to avoid hemorrhage.

HEPATIC ENCEPHALOPATHY
HEPATIC COMA

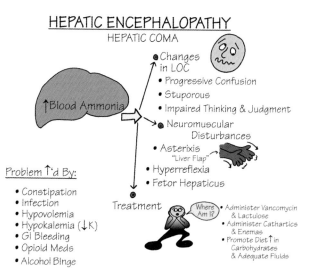

↑Blood Ammonia

- Changes in LOC
  - Progressive Confusion
  - Stuporous
  - Impaired Thinking & Judgment
- Neuromuscular Disturbances
  - Asterixis "Liver Flap"
  - Hyperreflexia
  - Fetor Hepaticus

Problem ↑'d By:

- Constipation
- Infection
- Hypovolemia
- Hypokalemia (↓K)
- GI Bleeding
- Opioid Meds
- Alcohol Binge

Treatment   Where Am I?
- Administer Vancomycin & Lactulose
- Administer Cathartics & Enemas
- Promote Diet ↑ in Carbohydrates & Adequate Fluids

What You Need to Know
Hepatic Encephalopathy

DEFINITION

Hepatic encephalopathy (HE) results from the inability of the liver to detoxify ammonia. It is a common complication of liver disease.

RISK FACTORS

- Can occur after placement of a transjugular intrahepatic portal-systemic shunt

COMPLICATIONS

- Hepatic coma → death

RECOGNIZE AND ANALYZE CUES

- Grading scale system used to classify the stages of HE
  - Uses three areas—level of consciousness, intellectual function, neurologic findings
  - Stage 0—minimal symptoms
  - Stage 1—mild symptoms, sleep problems, attention deficit
  - Stage 2—moderate symptoms, lethargy, disorientation, asterixis
  - Stage 3—severe symptoms, confusion, speech problems, asterixis
  - Stage 4—hepatic coma, no asterixis

MEDICAL MANAGEMENT: GENERATE SOLUTIONS

- Drugs: antibiotics (rifaximin), lactulose

NURSING MANAGEMENT: TAKE ACTION

1. Assess for changes in level of orientation, asterixis.
2. Evaluate serum ammonia levels daily.
3. Decrease the production of ammonia.
   - ↑carbohydrates and fluids (as tolerated).
   - ↓activity because ammonia is a by-product of metabolism.
   - Treat gastrointestinal bleeding because it ↑ammonia levels.
   - Avoid constipation because it ↑ammonia levels.
   - Administer lactulose; therapy must be titrated, as diarrhea may occur (monitor for hypokalemia).

HEPATITIS

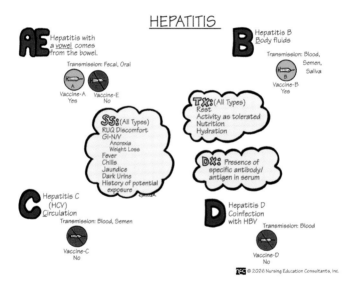

AE Hepatitis with a <u>vowel</u> comes from the bowel.

Transmission: Fecal, Oral

Vaccine-A — Yes
Vaccine-E — No

B Hepatitis B <u>B</u>ody fluids

Transmission: Blood, Semen, Saliva

Vaccine-B — Yes

SS: (All Types)
RUQ Discomfort
GI-N/V
   Anorexia
   Weight Loss
Fever
Chills
Jaundice
Dark Urine
History of potential exposure

TX: (All Types)
Rest
Activity as tolerated
Nutrition
Hydration

DX: Presence of specific antibody/antigen in serum

C Hepatitis C (HCV) <u>C</u>irculation

Transmission: Blood, Semen

Vaccine-C — No

D Hepatitis D Coinfection with HBV

Transmission: Blood

Vaccine-D — No

===================== **What You Need to Know** =====================
Hepatitis

DEFINITION

Hepatitis is a widespread inflammation of liver tissue with the most common cause being a viral infection. There are five categories of viruses—hepatitis A virus (HAV), hepatitis B virus (HBV), hepatitis C virus (HCV), hepatitis D virus (HDV), and hepatitis E virus (HEV).

MODE OF TRANSMISSION

- HAV—fecal-oral (primarily fecal contamination and oral ingestion)
- HBV—percutaneous (parenteral) or mucosal exposure to blood or blood products, sexual contact, perinatal transmission
- HCV—percutaneous (parenteral) or mucosal exposure to blood or blood products, sexual contact, perinatal contact
- HDV—HBV must precede HDV; chronic carriers of HBV always at risk
- HEV—fecal-oral (outbreaks associated with contaminated water supply in developing countries); uncommon in the United States

COMPLICATIONS

- Chronic hepatitis (HBV, HCV), cirrhosis, liver cancer
- Acute liver failure

RECOGNIZE AND ANALYZE CUES

- Regardless of the type of hepatitis, the clinical picture is similar.
- Diagnostic: testing for specific antibody or antigen; ↑alanine aminotransferase, ↑aspartate aminotransferase (AST), ↑serum bilirubin; ultrasound elastography (e.g., FibroScan); FibroTest (biomarker that uses the results of serum tests to assess the extent of hepatic fibrosis).

MEDICAL MANAGEMENT: GENERATE SOLUTIONS

- Preventive immunizations (HAV, HBV); postexposure prophylaxis—immune globulin (HAV), hepatitis B immune globulin
- Drugs (chronic hepatitis; HBV, HCV): immune modulator (pegylated interferon), nucleoside and nucleotide analogs, direct-acting antivirals for HCV

NURSING MANAGEMENT: TAKE ACTION

1. Understand transmission and preventive measures for all types of hepatitis.
2. Provide a well-balanced diet, vitamin supplements (B complex, K), avoid alcohol and drugs detoxified by the liver.
3. Encourage rest.

HEPATITIS A & E

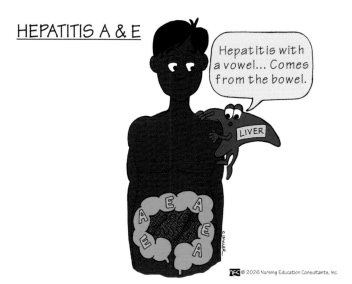

What You Need to Know
Hepatitis A and E

DEFINITION

Hepatitis A (HAV) and Hepatitis E (HEV) are types of hepatitis that have a fecal-oral mode of transmission. The mnemonic, "hepatitis with a *vowel*, comes from the *bowel*," can help you remember the fecal-oral transmission.

RISK FACTORS

- HAV—poor hygiene, improper food handling, homelessness, crowded situations, poor sanitary conditions
- HBV—living with chronically HBV-infected persons, patients on hemodialysis, healthcare personnel, public safety workers, blood product recipients, patients with organ and tissue transplantation, prisoners, veterans, homelessness

RECOGNIZE AND ANALYZE CUES

- Onset of HAV is more acute; symptoms are generally less severe
  - HAV in feces 1 to 2 weeks before the onset of symptoms, at least 1 week after the onset of illness, which means it can be carried and transmitted by persons who have undetectable infection
- Onset of HBV is more insidious; symptoms are more severe
  - Blood borne, sexual contact, perinatal transmission
  - Hepatitis carriers (patients who do not develop immunity after the infection) can infect others even though they are not sick and have no obvious signs of HBV

NURSING MANAGEMENT: TAKE ACTION

1. Anticipate the most patients will be carried for at home.
   - Nutrition therapy, avoid alcohol and hepatoxic meds.
   - Rest with gradual increase in activity.
2. Monitor for complications—bleeding tendencies, chronic hepatitis (HBV), cirrhosis, liver cancer.
3. Teach about regular follow-ups for at least 1 year after the diagnosis of hepatitis.

Important nursing interventions	Serious/life-threatening implications
Common signs & symptoms	Patient teaching

CHOLECYSTITIS

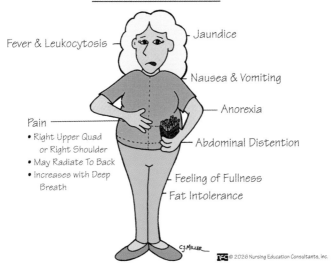

Fever & Leukocytosis

Jaundice

Nausea & Vomiting

Anorexia

Pain
- Right Upper Quad or Right Shoulder
- May Radiate To Back
- Increases with Deep Breath

Abdominal Distention

Feeling of Fullness

Fat Intolerance

What You Need to Know
Cholecystitis

DEFINITION

Cholecystitis is an inflammation of the gallbladder, which is frequently associated with obstruction caused by stones and may be acute or chronic.

RISK FACTORS

- Bile stasis, obesity
- Adhesions, cancer, anesthesia, opioids

COMPLICATIONS

- Gangrenous cholecystitis, subphrenic abscess, pancreatitis, cholangitis (inflammation of biliary ducts), biliary cirrhosis, fistulas, rupture of the gallbladder → peritonitis

RECOGNIZE AND ANALYZE CUES

- Onset may be sudden with severe steady pain (biliary colic); exacerbated by deep breathing
- Abdominal guarding, rigidity, fever
- Diagnostics: ↑white blood cells, ↑serum bilirubin, ↑liver enzymes (AST, lactate dehydrogenase); ultrasound, HIDA scan

MEDICAL MANAGEMENT: GENERATE SOLUTIONS

- Drugs: analgesics, anticholinergics, antibiotics
- Surgery: laparoscopic or open cholecystectomy
- Diet: ↓fat

NURSING MANAGEMENT: TAKE ACTION

1. Administer medications during acute attack (biliary colic).
2. Provide preoperative and postoperative care.
   - Modified left lateral recumbent position with right knee flexed to facilitate the movement of CO_2 gas pocket away from the diaphragm (lap chole).
   - May have a T-tube postoperative—maintain gravity drainage; do not clamp or irrigate.
3. Encourage a ↓low fat, ↑fiber, ↑calcium diet; eating small, more frequent meals.
4. Teach to avoid heavy lifting for 4 to 6 weeks (open chole).

Important nursing interventions	Serious/life-threatening implications
Common signs & symptoms	Patient teaching

LAPAROSCOPIC VS OPEN CHOLECYSTECTOMY

Laparoscopic

- Called a "lap chole."
- Ambulatory or same day surgery.
- Minimally invasive endoscopic surgery.
  - Involves 3–4 small incisions.
  - Abdominal cavity insufflated with 3–4 L of CO_2.
  - Referred shoulder discomfort from CO_2.
  - Minimal postoperative pain.
  - Glue, BANDAIDS, or Steri-strips cover tiny incisions.
- Teach patient to slowly add fat back into diet.
- Complications seldom occur.
- Death rate very low.

..VS..

Open Cholecystectomy (Traditional)

- Abdominal laparatomy.
- Removal of gall bladder through a right subcostal incision.
- May have a Jackson-Pratt (JP) drain.
- T-Tube may be inserted into common bile duct during surgery.
- Postoperative care.
- Encourage coughing, turning, deep breathing
- Diet progression: clear liquids, full liquids, soft, regular.
- Prevent respiratory complications due to position of incision area often prevents patient from deep breathing, etc.

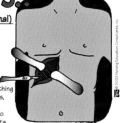

What You Need to Know

Laparoscopic Versus Open Cholecystectomy

DEFINITION

There are two primary surgical procedures for removing the gallbladder—a laparoscopic cholecystectomy (lap chole) and an open cholecystectomy (open chole or incisional chole).

COMPLICATIONS

- Hemorrhage, infection, injury to small bowel
- Lap chole: injury to common bile duct

LAPAROSCOPIC CHOLECYSTECTOMY

- Usually the treatment of choice.
  - Patient recovery is quicker; less postoperative pain.
- Gallbladder is removed through one to four small punctures in the abdomen.
- CO_2 gas is passed into the abdomen to expand the area.
  - May have referred shoulder and chest discomfort postoperatively.

OPEN CHOLECYSTECTOMY

- Removal of the gallbladder through a right subcostal incision.
- May have a T-tube placed in the common bile duct.
  - Do not irrigate or clamp; do not raise above the level of the gallbladder.
  - Observe for bile drainage around the tube.
  - Drainage—bloody initially, then greenish brown.
  - Drainage around 500 mL/day for several days after surgery; drainage gradually decreases → tube removed.

NURSING MANAGEMENT: TAKE ACTION

1. Teach postoperative care after lap chole.
   - Remove the bandages on the puncture sites the day after surgery, then it is okay to shower.
   - Notify healthcare provider (HCP) about: redness, swelling, bile-colored drainage or pus from any incision, severe abdominal pain, nausea, vomiting, fever, chills.
   - Return to work within 1 week of surgery.
   - Resume normal diet; may tolerate a ↓fat diet initially.
2. Teach postoperative care after an open chole.
   - Monitor for respiratory problems.
   - Notify HCP about: redness, swelling, bile-colored drainage or pus from incision, severe abdominal pain, nausea, vomiting, fever, chills.
   - Avoid heavy lifting for 4 to 6 weeks.
   - May tolerate a ↓fat diet initially.

PANCREATITIS
(Inflammatory Condition of the Pancreas)

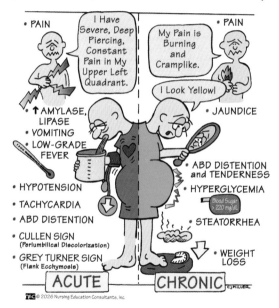

What You Need to Know
Pancreatitis

DEFINITION

Pancreatitis is an inflammatory condition of the pancreas. There are two types: acute (can be life threatening) and chronic pancreatitis.

RISK FACTORS

- Biliary tract obstructive disease
- Hyperlipidemia, chronic alcohol use

COMPLICATIONS

- Pancreatic pseudocyst or abscess
- Pleural effusion, atelectasis, pneumonia, acute respiratory distress syndrome

RECOGNIZE AND ANALYZE CUES

- Acute: abdominal pain, nausea, vomiting, low-grade fever, leukocytosis, hypotension, tachycardia, jaundice
- Chronic: abdominal pain, weight loss, constipation, mild jaundice with dark urine, steatorrhea, diabetes

MEDICAL MANAGEMENT: GENERATE SOLUTIONS

- Drugs: opioid analgesic (morphine), proton pump inhibitor (omeprazole), antibiotics (if necrotizing pancreatitis); insulin and enzymes (pancrelipase) for chronic pancreatitis

NURSING MANAGEMENT: TAKE ACTION

Acute pancreatitis:
1. Monitor for respiratory distress.
   - Listen to lung sounds and monitor O_2 saturation on a regular basis.
2. Administer analgesics for pain.
3. Maintain NPO status; IV fluids, nasogastric suction.
4. Maintain bed rest; diet (if not NPO) ↓fat, ↑carbohydrate.

Chronic pancreatitis:
1. Teach about pain management, diet, pancreatic enzyme replacement, and diabetes control to manage pancreatic insufficiency.
   - Small, bland, frequent meals—↓fat to decrease pancreatic stimulation.
2. Teach to avoid consuming alcohol and caffeinated beverages.

INCREASED INTRACRANIAL PRESSURE

- Changes in LOC
  - Flattening of Affect
  - ↓Orientation & Attention
  - Coma

- Eyes
  - Papilledema
  - Pupillary Changes
  - Impaired Eye Movement

- Posturing
  - Decerebrate
  - Decorticate
  - Flaccid

- Decreased Motor Function
  - Change in Motor Ability
  - Posturing

- Headache

- Seizures
  - Impaired Sensory & Motor Function

- Changes in Vital Signs: Cushing Triad
  - ↑Systolic BP "Widening Pulse Pressure"
  - ↓Pulse
  - Irregular Resp Pattern

- Vomiting
  - Not Preceded by Nausea
  - May be Projectile

- Changes in Speech

- Infants:
  - Bulging Fontanels
  - Cranial Suture Separation
  - ↑Head Circumference
  - High Pitched Cry

— What You Need to Know —
Increased Intracranial Pressure

DEFINITION

An increase in intracranial pressure (IICP) occurs when there is an increase in the size or amount of intracranial contents. Because the cranial vault is rigid, there is minimal room for expansion of the intracranial components. This is potentially life threatening.

RISK FACTORS

- ↑intracranial blood volume (vasodilation, bleeding)
- ↑cerebrospinal fluid (CSF)
- ↑in bulk of brain tissue (cerebral edema)

COMPLICATIONS

- CSF leaks (especially with a basilar skull fracture)
- Herniation (shifting of intracranial contents from one compartment to another → brain ischemia → death)
- Permanent brain damage

RECOGNIZE AND ANALYZE CUES

- Review figure

MEDICAL MANAGEMENT: GENERATE SOLUTIONS

- Drugs: osmotic diuretic (mannitol), IV hypertonic saline (↓IICP), antiseizure drugs (phenytoin), corticosteroids (for brain tumors, bacterial meningitis), H_2 receptor antagonist (cimetidine), proton pump inhibitor (pantoprazole), or barbiturates (↓cerebral metabolism)
- ICP monitoring: ventriculostomy

NURSING MANAGEMENT: TAKE ACTION

Patient will be treated in intensive care unit.

1. Elevate head of the bed to 30 degrees—head in neutral position.
2. Anticipate mechanical ventilation, ICP monitoring, cerebral oxygenation monitoring.
3. Frequent bedside neurochecks, Glasgow coma scale.
4. Maintain fluid balance; assess osmolality.
5. Maintain systolic arterial pressure between 100 and 160 mm Hg.

INCREASED INTRACRANIAL PRESSURE (IICP)—
CUSHING TRIAD
(Symptoms of IICP Are Opposite of Shock)

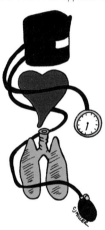

* IICP *

↑Systolic B/P
↓Pulse
↓Respirations

* Shock *

↓B/P
↑Pulse
↑Respirations

Increased Intracranial Pressure—Cushing Triad

DEFINITION

Cushing triad signs are a medical emergency and indicate brainstem compression and impending death. It is characterized by systolic hypertension with a widening pulse pressure, bradycardia with a full and bounding pulse, and irregular respirations. *Symptoms are opposite of shock.*

RISK FACTORS

- Brain mass (hematoma, contusion, abscess, tumor)
- Cerebral edema (associated with brain tumors, hydrocephalus, head injury, brain inflammation [meningitis])

COMPLICATIONS

- Inadequate cerebral perfusion
- Cerebral herniation—brain tissue forced from a compartment of greater pressure to compartment of less pressure
- Tentorial herniation (central herniation)—brain herniates downward through brainstem (foramen magnum)
- Uncal herniation occurs when there is lateral and downward herniation
- Cingulate herniation occurs when there is lateral displacement of brain tissue beneath the falx cerebri (thin wall of dura that folds down between the two cortexes)

RECOGNIZE AND ANALYZE CUES

- Changes in the level of consciousness
  - Most sensitive, reliable indicator of neuro status
- Vital signs—Cushing triad
- Dilation of pupils
  - Compression of oculomotor nerve → pupil dilation on the same side (ipsilateral)
  - Papilledema (edema of optic disc)
  - Fixed, unilateral, dilated pupil indicates brain herniation
- Decline in motor function—decorticate (flexor posturing), decerebrate (extensor posturing; indicates more serious damage)
- Headache
- Vomiting (projectile, without nausea)
- Diagnostics: CT scan, MRI, electroencephalography, cerebral angiography, ICP and brain tissue measurement, brain tissue oxygenation measurement, positron emission tomography, transcranial Doppler studies, evoked potential studies

SEIZURES

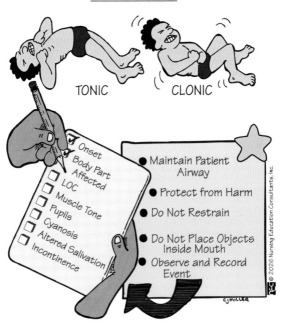

TONIC CLONIC

- Onset
- Body Part Affected
- ☐ LOC
- ☐ Muscle Tone
- ☐ Pupils
- ☐ Cyanosis
- ☐ Altered Salivation
- ☐ Incontinence

- Maintain Patient Airway
- Protect from Harm
- Do Not Restrain
- Do Not Place Objects Inside Mouth
- Observe and Record Event

What You Need to Know
Seizures

DEFINITION

A seizure is a sudden, uncontrolled electrical discharge of neurons in the brain that interrupts normal function. Seizure disorder, or epilepsy, is a group of neurological diseases marked by recurrent seizures.

RISK FACTORS

- Congenital brain malformations, CNS infections
- Head trauma, stroke, tumors, fever
- Acute alcohol withdrawal, substance abuse

COMPLICATIONS

- Status epilepticus: state of continuous seizure activity
- Sudden unexpected death in epilepsy

RECOGNIZE AND ANALYZE CUES

- Generalized onset seizures
  - Tonic-clonic (formerly called grand mal): most common type for this category; *tonic phase*: sudden loss of consciousness, stiffening of body; *clonic phase*: rhythmic contractions of all four extremities; *postictal phase*: headache, confusion, fatigue, often no memory of seizure
  - Absence: impaired awareness and responsiveness; occurs in children most often
  - Atonic or *drop attack*: abrupt loss of muscle tone
  - Myoclonic: repetitive muscle contractions
- Focal onset seizures (may be motor or nonmotor)
  - With retained awareness (previously called simple partial seizures); can present with auras and postictal phase; have unusual feelings or sensations
  - With impaired awareness (previously called complex partial seizures): most common type of seizure in adults with epilepsy. Can stare into space, motionless, dream-like state, or engage in automatisms, then enters postictal phase
- Psychogenic nonepileptic seizures: triggered by emotional events not neuronal activity

MEDICAL MANAGEMENT: GENERATE SOLUTIONS

- Drugs: antiseizure
- Surgery: if unresponsive to drug therapy

STROKE
(Brain Attack, CVA)

- Headache
- Mental Changes
  - Confusion
  - Disorientation
  - Memory Impairment
- Aphasia ($\frac{\text{CVA Left}}{\text{Hemisphere}}$)
- Resp Problems
  (↓Neuromuscular Control)
  - ↓Cough/Swallow
    Reflex
- Agnosia (↓$\frac{\text{Sensory}}{\text{Interpretation}}$)
- Incontinence
- Seizures

- Hemiparesis or Hemiplegia
- Emotional Lability
- Visual Changes
  (Homonymous Hemianopsia)

- Diplopia, Ptosis, and Loss
  of Corneal Reflex
- Vomiting
- Spatial-Perceptual Defects
  (CVA Right Hemisphere)
- Hypertension
- Apraxia
  (↓Learned Movements)

Transient Ischemic
Attack (TIA):
- Confusion
- Vertigo
- Dysarthria
- Transient Hemiparesis
- Temporary Vision
  Changes
- Typically Lasts Less
  Than 1 Hour

Focal Neurological S & S:
- Paralysis
- Sensory Loss
- Language Disorder
- Reflex Changes

© 2026 Nursing Education Consultants, Inc.

What You Need to Know
Stroke Symptoms

DEFINITION

Stroke, or brain attack, is the disruption of the blood supply to an area of the brain, resulting in ischemia, tissue necrosis, and sudden loss of brain function. *Transient ischemic attack* (TIA) is a transient episode of neurologic dysfunction caused by focal brain, spinal cord, or retinal ischemia, but without acute infarction of the brain. Symptoms typically last less than 1 hour.

RISK FACTORS

- Nonmodifiable
  - Age, sex, race, family history/genetics, prior stroke or TIA
- Modifiable
  - Metabolic: diabetes, dyslipidemia, obesity, metabolic syndrome
  - Lifestyle: smoking, alcohol, cocaine/amphetamine use, physical inactivity, poor diet
  - Cardiovascular: hypertension, atrial fibrillation, valvular heart disease, endocarditis, recent myocardial infarction
  - Sleep apnea

RECOGNIZE AND ANALYZE CUES

- Review figure
- Affects motor activity, bladder and bowel function, intellect, spatial perception, personality, affect, sensation, swallowing, communication
  - Area and functions affected are related to the artery involved and area of the brain it supplies
  - Symptoms relate to right-brain damage and left-brain damage (see notecards, Left CVA and Right CVA)

MEDICAL MANAGEMENT: GENERATE SOLUTIONS

- Thrombolysis, IV administration of tPA
  - Door-to-needle time of <60 minutes
  - Neurologic exams every 15 minutes during infusion, every 30 minutes for the next 6 hours, then hourly until 24 hours after treatment
  - Measure BP every 15 minutes for first 2 hours, every 30 minutes for next 6 hours, then every hour until 24 hours after treatment; maintain BP <185/105 mm Hg

FAST RECOGNITION OF A STROKE

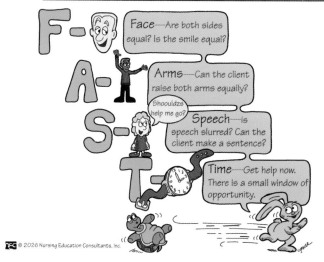

What You Need to Know
FAST Recognition of a Stroke

DEFINITION

FAST is an acronym to help recognize the symptoms of a stroke. The acronym FAST (**F**acial drooping, **A**rm weakness, **S**peech difficulties, and **T**ime) has been used by the National Stroke Association, American Heart Association, and others to educate the public on detecting symptoms of a stroke. When these signs are noted, it is important to call 911.

TYPES OF STROKE

- Ischemic (occlusive)
  - Thrombotic: atherosclerotic narrowing of the cerebral artery with plaque rupture causing clot formation
    (1) Associated with hypertension and diabetes
    (2) Most common cause of stroke
  - Embolic: occlusion of a cerebral artery by an embolus from another part of the body
    (1) Second most common cause of stroke
    (2) Common site of origin is the heart
    (3) May affect any age group; sudden onset of symptoms
- Hemorrhagic: bleeding into brain tissue, subarachnoid space, or ventricles
  - Blood forms clot causing increased pressure on brain tissue
  - Subarachnoid bleed irritates meningeal tissue and may cause vasospasm and ↓blood flow to brain

RECOGNIZE AND ANALYZE CUES

- In addition to FAST, report the sudden onset of the following:
  - Confusion
  - Numbness or weakness, especially on one side of the body
  - Severe headache with no known cause
  - Trouble seeing in one or both eyes, double vision
  - Trouble walking, dizziness, loss of balance or coordination

---

| Important nursing interventions | Serious/life-threatening implications |
| Common signs & symptoms | Patient teaching |

LEFT CVA

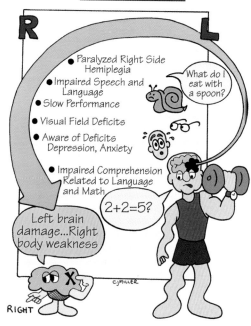

What You Need to Know
Left CVA

DEFINITION

A left CVA is left brain hemisphere damage (stroke on the left side of the brain) and involves motor deficits on the right side of the body. The left brain hemisphere is the dominant hemisphere in most patients and is the center for speech, language, mathematic skills, and analytic thinking.

RECOGNIZE AND ANALYZE CUES

- Hemiplegia (paralysis) or hemiparesis (partial weakness) on body's right side
- Cognitive impairments: deficit in memory or problem-solving ability; slow performance; cautious
- Aphasia: speaking and language impairment
- Dysarthria: problem with pronunciation, articulation, and phonation due to muscular control of speech
- Apraxia of speech: difficulty in putting words together in correct order while speaking
- Dysphagia: difficulty in swallowing
- Homonymous hemianopia: sees one-half of their expected field of vision in each eye (e.g., loss of vision in right field of each eye)
- Memory loss
- Aware of deficits; depression, anxiety

Important nursing interventions	Serious/life-threatening implications
Common signs & symptoms	Patient teaching

RIGHT CVA

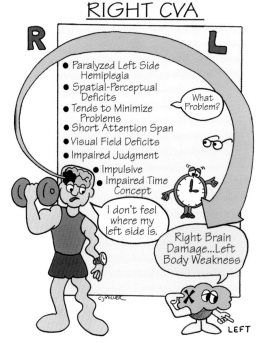

R   L

- Paralyzed Left Side Hemiplegia
- Spatial-Perceptual Deficits
- Tends to Minimize Problems
- Short Attention Span
- Visual Field Deficits
- Impaired Judgment
- Impulsive
- Impaired Time Concept

What Problem?

I don't feel where my left side is.

Right Brain Damage...Left Body Weakness

LEFT

© 2026 Nursing Education Consultants, Inc.

What You Need to Know
Right CVA

DEFINITION

A right CVA is right brain hemisphere damage (stroke on the right side of the brain) and involves motor deficits on the left side of the body. The right brain hemisphere is more involved with visual and spatial awareness and proprioception (sense of body position). A person who has a right CVA is often unaware of any deficits, may be disoriented to time and place, and have poor judgment.

RECOGNIZE AND ANALYZE CUES

- Hemiplegia (paralysis) or hemiparesis (partial weakness) on body's left side
- Left spatial neglect: experience an unawareness of the left side of their environment
  - Does not see objects on left side and may bump into them
  - Does not comprehend body parts or objects on the left side
  - Does not see words on the left side of a page of paper
- Homonymous hemianopia: sees one-half of their expected field of vision in each eye (e.g., loss of vision in left field of each eye)
- Personality changes
  - Sudden, uncontrollable outbursts of laughing or crying; impulsive
  - Inappropriate child-like behavior
  - Flattened affect
- Short attention span, rapid performance
- Difficulty in recognizing faces, memory loss
- Denies or minimizes problems
- Impaired judgment and time concepts

Important nursing interventions	Serious/life-threatening implications
Common signs & symptoms	Patient teaching

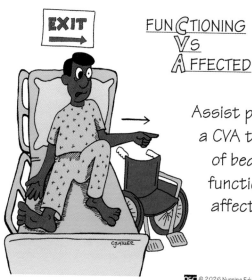

FUNCTIONING Vs AFFECTED

Assist patient with a CVA to get out of bed on the functioning vs. affected side.

What You Need to Know
CVA—Functioning VS Affected

DEFINITION

The acronym "FUNCTIONING **V**S **A**FFECTED" can help in remembering to assist the patient with a CVA to get out of bed on their functioning side versus their affected (hemiplegic or hemiparesis) side.

NURSING MANAGEMENT: TAKE ACTION

1. Place client in a side-lying position with the head elevated; keep NPO status until swallow evaluation.
2. If unconscious, use the oropharyngeal airway to prevent airway obstruction by the tongue.
3. Cough and deep breathe for every 2 hours (q2h).
4. Need swallow evaluation before initiating oral feedings.
   - Maintain high-Fowler position for feeding.
   - Administer oral feedings cautiously; check gag and swallowing reflexes before feeding.
   - Place food on unaffected side of mouth.
   - Select foods that are easy to control in the mouth (thick liquids) and easy to swallow; thin liquids often promote coughing.
5. Passive range of motion (ROM) on affected side; active ROM on unaffected side.
6. Legs neutral position; prevent external rotation of affected hip; place trochanter roll or rolled pillow at thigh; prevent foot drop.
7. Reposition q2h; limit time spent on affected side.
   - Protect affected side: do not give injections on that side; watch for pressure areas.
8. Maintain affected arm in neutral (slightly flexed) position with each joint slightly higher than preceding one.
9. Assist the client out of bed on the unaffected side because it provides stabilization and balance.

Important nursing interventions

Common signs & symptoms

Serious/life-threatening implications

Patient teaching

SPINAL CORD INJURY

(Paralysis Below The Level of Injury)

Injuries ↑C4 = Paralysis of
respiratory muscles AND
all four extremities.
(Tetraplegia Formerly Called Quadriplegia)

Higher the injury
Greater the loss
of function.

Temperature Regulation
Problems ↓Level
of Injury...

"SNAP!" "SNAP!"

© 2026 Nursing Education Consultants, Inc.

What You Need to Know
Spinal Cord Injury

DEFINITION

Spinal cord injury (SCI) is damage to the spinal cord, generally a result of trauma. The degree of injury is classified as complete, resulting in loss of both sensory and motor function below the level of injury, or incomplete, with some sensation or motor function below the level of injury.

RISK FACTORS

- Trauma: falls, acts of violence (usually gunshot wounds), sports or recreation-related accidents (diving into shallow water)

COMPLICATIONS

- Spinal shock (occurs immediately)
- Neurogenic (vasogenic) shock

RECOGNIZE AND ANALYZE CUES

- Injury from C1 to T1; paralysis of all four extremities → tetraplegia (formerly called quadriplegia)
- Paraplegia (paralysis and loss of sensation in the legs) SCI level of T2↓

MEDICAL MANAGEMENT: GENERATE SOLUTIONS

- Emergency intervention required; stabilize cervical spine, manage airway, breathing, circulation
- Immobilization of the vertebral column in cervical fracture
- Spinal surgery to decompress spinal cord and stabilize spine

NURSING MANAGEMENT: TAKE ACTION

1. Immobilize and stabilize vertebral column.
2. Assess ABCs (airway, breathing, circulation); anticipate intubation.
3. Provide O_2 by high-humidity mask.
4. Treat spinal shock.
5. Administer medications, for example, atropine for heart rate; dopamine for blood pressure (BP) to maintain systolic BP >90 mm Hg, mean arterial pressure >85.
6. Administer IV fluids; insert urinary catheter.
7. Insert NG tube; attach to suction.
8. Assess nutrition; provide therapeutic diet.
9. Maintain normal body temperature.
10. Provide pain management.
11. Provide VTE and stress ulcer prophylaxis; prevent pressure injury.
12. Provide bowel and bladder retraining.
13. Assess for autonomic dysreflexia (AD).

AUTONOMIC DYSREFLEXIA

(Spinal Cord Injury At T-6 Or Higher)

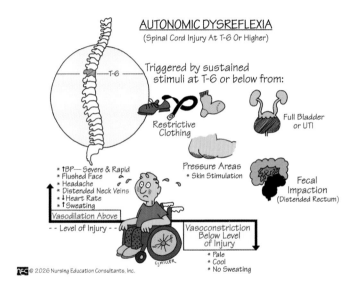

T-6

Triggered by sustained stimuli at T-6 or below from:

Restrictive Clothing

Full Bladder or UTI

Pressure Areas
* Skin Stimulation

Fecal Impaction
(Distended Rectum)

* ↑BP— Severe & Rapid
* Flushed Face
* Headache
* Distended Neck Veins
* ↓ Heart Rate
* ↑ Sweating

Vasodilation Above

- - Level of Injury - -

Vasoconstriction Below Level of Injury
* Pale
* Cool
* No Sweating

CJMILLER

Neurology

What You Need to Know
Autonomic Dysreflexia

DEFINITION

Autonomic dysreflexia (AD) is a potentially life-threatening condition in which noxious visceral or cutaneous stimuli cause a sudden, massive, uninhibited reflex sympathetic discharge in T-6 injury or higher SCI.

RISK FACTORS

- Distended bladder or rectum (most common precipitating cause)
- Skin stimulation, tight clothing

COMPLICATIONS

- Severe hypertension → death

RECOGNIZE AND ANALYZE CUES

- Hypertension, bradycardia, sudden, pounding headache
- Nausea, restlessness, piloerection (i.e., goosebumps), flushing and sweating above SCI level, blurred vision
- Pale, cool extremities, no sweating below SCI level

NURSING MANAGEMENT: TAKE ACTION

1. Elevate the head of the bed; check BP.
2. Assess for sources of stimuli: distended bladder (check urinary tubing), fecal impaction, constipation, tight clothing.
3. Relieve the stimuli; dysreflexia will subside.
4. Maintain cardiovascular support during period of hypertension; administer short-acting antihypertensive as prescribed.
5. Anticipate hypertensive crisis from dysreflexia will require immediate intervention.
6. Initiate measures to ↓incidence of AD.
   - Maintain regular bowel function; monitor urine output.
   - Use local anesthetic when manual rectal stimulation is used to promote bowel function.
   - Teach to wear a Medic Alert bracelet.

Important nursing interventions	Serious/life-threatening implications
Common signs & symptoms	Patient teaching

PARKINSON DISEASE

- Onset usually gradual, after age 50.
  (Slowly progressive)

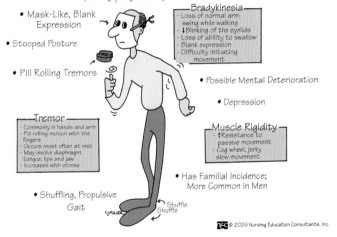

- Mask-Like, Blank Expression
- Stooped Posture
- Pill Rolling Tremors

Bradykinesia
- Loss of normal arm swing while walking
- ↓Blinking of the eyelids
- Loss of ability to swallow
- Blank expression
- Difficulty initiating movement

- Possible Mental Deterioration
- Depression

Tremor
- Commonly in hands and arm
- Pill rolling motion with the fingers
- Occurs most often at rest
- May involve diaphragm, tongue, lips and jaw
- Increases with stress

Muscle Rigidity
- ↑Resistance to passive movement
- Cog wheel, jerky slow movement

- Has Familial Incidence; More Common in Men
- Shuffling, Propulsive Gait

Shuffle
Shuffle

What You Need to Know
Parkinson Disease

DEFINITION

Parkinson disease is a progressive neurodegenerative disorder with the gradual onset characterized by slowness in the initiation and execution of movement (bradykinesia), increased muscle tone (rigidity), tremor at rest, and gait changes.

RISK FACTORS

- Traumatic brain injury, brain tumor
- Family history; male, >40 years of age

COMPLICATIONS

- Dysphagia, malnutrition, dementia, ↑fall risk
- Dyskinesias (spontaneous involuntary movements)

RECOGNIZE AND ANALYZE CUES

- Shaky (pill-rolling tremor at rest), stiff (cogwheel rigidity), freezing
- Slow (bradykinesia), stumbling (shuffling gait, postural instability)
- Masklike facial expression

MEDICAL MANAGEMENT: GENERATE SOLUTIONS

- Drugs: antiparkinson (dopaminergic or anticholinergic)
- Deep brain stimulation—electrodes implanted in brain, connected to a pulse generator that delivers electrical current to alleviate symptoms; most common treatment
- Stereotactic pallidotomy (tissue ablation)

NURSING MANAGEMENT: TAKE ACTION

1. Maintain safety; high risk for falls; monitor for orthostatic hypotension.
2. Maintain nutrition; monitor for difficulty swallowing.
   - ↑calories and protein; provide easily chewed foods.
   - Frequent small meals; allow ample time for eating.
3. Maintain muscle function; active/passive ROM to extremities.
4. Promote physical, occupational, speech therapy as indicated.
5. Teach importance of physical exercise and well-balanced diet.

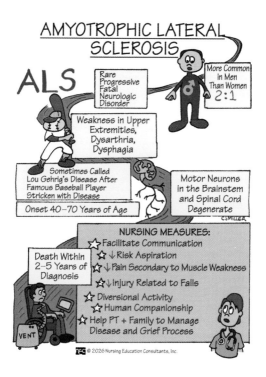

AMYOTROPHIC LATERAL SCLEROSIS

ALS

Rare Progressive Fatal Neurologic Disorder

More Common in Men Than Women 2:1

Weakness in Upper Extremities, Dysarthria, Dysphagia

Sometimes Called Lou Gehrig's Disease After Famous Baseball Player Stricken with Disease

Onset 40-70 Years of Age

Motor Neurons in the Brainstem and Spinal Cord Degenerate

NURSING MEASURES:
☆ Facilitate Communication
☆ ↓ Risk Aspiration
☆ ↓ Pain Secondary to Muscle Weakness
☆ ↓ Injury Related to Falls
☆ Diversional Activity
☆ Human Companionship
☆ Help PT + Family to Manage Disease and Grief Process

Death Within 2-5 Years of Diagnosis

VENT

What You Need to Know
Amyotrophic Lateral Sclerosis

DEFINITION

Amyotrophic lateral sclerosis (ALS), also known as Lou Gehrig disease, is a rare, progressive, invariably fatal degeneration of motor neurons. Causes are unknown, and there is no cure. Death occurs within 2 to 5 years (usually from respiratory failure).

RISK FACTORS

- Family history
- Age >40 years and <70 years
- More common in males

RECOGNIZE AND ANALYZE CUES

- Progressive muscle weakness and atrophy (classic signs); death
- Diagnostics: MRI of brain

MEDICAL MANAGEMENT: GENERATE SOLUTIONS

- Drugs: riluzole, edaravone (slow progression)

NURSING MANAGEMENT: TAKE ACTION

1. Provide emotional support due to devastating physical nature of illness while the patient remains cognitively intact.
2. Palliative care for symptom management for end-of-life care.
3. Provide respite care and psychosocial support for family.

Important nursing interventions	Serious/life-threatening implications
Common signs & symptoms	Patient teaching

MULTIPLE SCLEROSIS

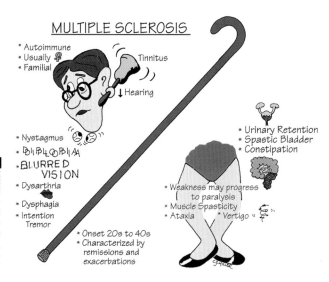

* Autoimmune
* Usually ♀
* Familial

Tinnitus

↓Hearing

* Nystagmus
* DIPLOPIA
* BLURRED VISION
* Dysarthria
* Dysphagia
* Intention Tremor

* Urinary Retention
* Spastic Bladder
* Constipation

* Weakness may progress to paralysis
* Muscle Spasticity
* Ataxia   * Vertigo

* Onset 20s to 40s
* Characterized by remissions and exacerbations

What You Need to Know
Multiple Sclerosis

DEFINITION

Multiple sclerosis is a chronic, unpredictable, progressive, degenerative disorder characterized by multiple areas of demyelination from inflammatory scarring of the myelin sheath surrounding neurons in the brain and spinal cord.

RISK FACTORS

- More common in females; onset age 20 to 40 years

COMPLICATIONS

- Infection (pulmonary due to immobility)

RECOGNIZE AND ANALYZE CUES

- Symptoms vary based on the area of CNS involved
- Review figure
- Diagnostics: delayed visual evoked potential (VEP)

MEDICAL MANAGEMENT: GENERATE SOLUTIONS

- Drugs: disease-modifying drugs—interferons, monoclonal antibodies (natalizumab), and synthetic agents; corticosteroids

NURSING MANAGEMENT: TAKE ACTION

1. Maintain adequate respiratory and urinary tract function.
2. Promote nutrition—food easy to chew; monitor swallowing reflex.
3. Maintain or improve muscle strength and mobility.
4. Encourage independence in ADLs.
5. Teach about lifestyle modifications.
   - Identify factors that trigger exacerbations (e.g., infection, trauma, life virus immunization, childbirth, stress, change in climate).
   - Initiate safety measures due to ↓sensation.

| Important nursing interventions | Serious/life-threatening implications |
| Common signs & symptoms | Patient teaching |

GUILLAIN-BARRÉ SYNDROME

Risk Factors:
- Possibly Autoimmune
- Association with Influenza Immunization
- Frequently preceded by mild respiratory or GI infection

- Progresses over hours to days
- Maximal Weakness Reached in 4 Weeks
- Minimal Muscle Atrophy

Venti-lator

E-T Tube

- Symmetrical Paralysis

Causes Problems With:
- Respiration
- Talking
- Swallowing
- Bowel & Bladder Function

Begins in lower extremities and ascends bilaterally
1) Weakness
2) Hypotonia and Areflexia
3) Bilateral Paresthesia Progressing to Paralysis
4) Pain—Worse at Night
5) Autonomic Disturbances—↑BP, ↓Pulse, Heart Block

What You Need to Know
Guillain-Barré Syndrome

DEFINITION

A rare, acute inflammatory, autoimmune disorder that causes acute peripheral neuropathy with ascending paralysis that progressively worsens for up to 4 weeks followed by a slow spontaneous recovery of function.

RISK FACTORS

- Respiratory or GI infection

COMPLICATIONS

- Respiratory failure → mechanical ventilation

RECOGNIZE AND ANALYZE CUES

- Weakness, paresthesia, hypotonia of limbs
- Pain, worse at night
- Paralysis of respiratory muscles

MEDICAL MANAGEMENT: GENERATE SOLUTIONS

- Supportive care—mechanical ventilation
- Plasma exchange (plasmapheresis), high-dose IV immunoglobulin (IVIG)

NURSING MANAGEMENT: TAKE ACTION

1. Evaluate rate of progress of paralysis; assess changes in respiratory pattern.
   - If ascending paralysis is rapid, prepare for endotracheal intubation and respiratory assistance.
2. Maintain NPO status if gag reflex is impaired.
3. Assess for involvement of the autonomic nervous system—orthostatic hypotension, ↓or ↑BP or pulse, cardiac dysrhythmias, urinary retention, paralytic ileus.

Important nursing interventions   Serious/life-threatening implications

Common signs & symptoms   Patient teaching

MYASTHENIA GRAVIS

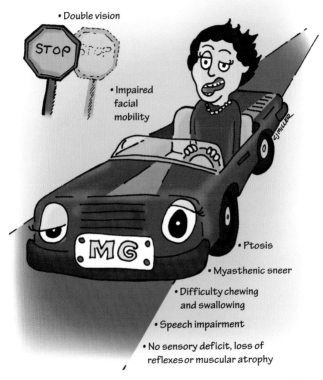

- Double vision
- Impaired facial mobility
- Ptosis
- Myasthenic sneer
- Difficulty chewing and swallowing
- Speech impairment
- No sensory deficit, loss of reflexes or muscular atrophy

What You Need to Know
Myasthenia Gravis

DEFINITION

Myasthenia gravis is a rare progressive autoimmune disease characterized by fluctuating muscle weakness because of impaired acetylcholine receptors.

EXACERBATION RISK FACTORS

- Fatigue, pregnancy, illness, trauma
- Temperature extremes, stress, hypokalemia

COMPLICATIONS

- Acute respiratory arrest, chronic respiratory insufficiency
- Myasthenic crisis—an acute worsening of symptoms

RECOGNIZE AND ANALYZE CUES

- Course is variable and characterized by exacerbations
- Diagnosis: electromyogram

MEDICAL MANAGEMENT: GENERATE SOLUTIONS

- Drugs: anticholinesterase (pyridostigmine), corticosteroids (prednisone), immunosuppressants (azathioprine, cyclosporine)
- Plasma electrophoresis (plasmapheresis), IVIG
- Surgery: removal of thymus (thymectomy)

NURSING MANAGEMENT: TAKE ACTION

1. Anticipate hospitalizations related to an acute myasthenic crisis, cholinergic crisis, or respiratory tract infection.
2. Distinguish between a myasthenic crisis and a cholinergic crisis.
   - Maintain adequate ventilatory support during crisis.
   - If myasthenic crisis occurs, neostigmine may be administered.
   - If cholinergic crisis occurs, atropine may be administered, and cholinergic medications may be reevaluated.
3. Avoid use of sedatives and tranquilizers; can cause respiratory depression.
4. Teach about the importance of taking medication on a regular basis; peak effect of the medication should coincide with mealtimes.
5. Teach about the need to wear an eye patch to protect cornea when ptosis is severe.
6. Teach about factors that can precipitate a myasthenic crisis—emotional upset, severe fatigue, infections, and exposure to extreme temperatures.

CHOLINERGIC CRISIS

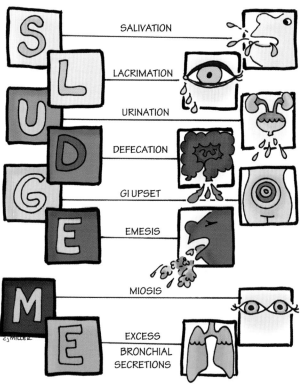

SALIVATION

LACRIMATION

URINATION

DEFECATION

GI UPSET

EMESIS

MIOSIS

EXCESS BRONCHIAL SECRETIONS

What You Need to Know
Cholinergic Crisis

DEFINITION

Cholinergic crisis is caused by substances that stimulate, enhance, or mimic the neurotransmitter acetylcholine, the primary neurotransmitter of the parasympathetic nervous systems. Acetylcholine stimulates two cholinergic, muscarinic, and nicotinic receptors. Muscarinic receptors work in both the peripheral and central nervous systems. Nicotinic receptors work in the central nervous system and at the neuromuscular junction. In addition, cholinergic crisis can be a toxic response to anticholinesterase medications, which necessitates anticholinesterase medications being withheld. This response is rare with proper dosing of pyridostigmine.

RISK FACTORS

- Overdose of anticholinesterase medications
- Organophosphate poisoning by nerve gases, pesticides, carbamate insecticides

COMPLICATIONS

- Bronchospasm, respiratory failure (due to weakness in respiratory muscles)
- Aspiration pneumonia (due to hypersalivation)
- Cardiovascular collapse → cardiac arrest → death

RECOGNIZE AND ANALYZE CUES

- Cholinergic crisis symptoms are very similar to myasthenic crisis
  - Inadequate dosing with an anticholinesterase causes a myasthenic crisis; excessive dosing causes a cholinergic crisis
- Involuntary muscle contraction, extreme weakness, flaccid muscle paralysis
- Sweating, excessive salivation, constricted pupils
- Nausea, vomiting, diarrhea, abdominal cramps

MEDICAL MANAGEMENT: GENERATE SOLUTIONS

- Drugs: atropine, pralidoxime
- Decontamination; need for personal protective equipment

NURSING MANAGEMENT: TAKE ACTION

1. Initiate care using the ABCDEs (airway, breathing, circulation, disability, exposure).
   - If condition due to organophosphate poisoning, remove clothing, wash skin and eyes.
   - If due to excessive anticholinesterase medication, withhold dose.
2. Healthcare workers should wear personal protective equipment to prevent dermal and inhalation exposure.

BELL PALSY

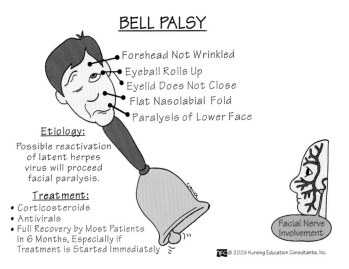

- Forehead Not Wrinkled
- Eyeball Rolls Up
- Eyelid Does Not Close
- Flat Nasolabial Fold
- Paralysis of Lower Face

Etiology:

Possible reactivation
of latent herpes
virus will proceed
facial paralysis.

Treatment:

- Corticosteroids
- Antivirals
- Full Recovery by Most Patients
  in 6 Months, Especially if
  Treatment is Started Immediately

Facial Nerve
Involvement

What You Need to Know
Bell Palsy

DEFINITION

Bell palsy is a transient disorder affecting the facial nerve (CN VII). Inflammation of CN VII causes a disruption of the motor branches on one side of the face, resulting in muscle weakness or flaccidity on the affected side.

RISK FACTORS

- Pregnancy, diabetes mellitus, obesity
- Upper respiratory infection, chronic hypertension
- Extremes of temperature

COMPLICATIONS

- Corneal abrasion or ulceration
- Residual effects of facial asymmetry, abnormal facial movements

RECOGNIZE AND ANALYZE CUES

- Cannot close eye, wrinkle forehead, smile, whistle, or grimace
- Tearing may stop or become excessive
- Face appears masklike sags

MEDICAL MANAGEMENT: GENERATE SOLUTIONS

- Drugs: early treatment (within 72 hours of onset) with corticosteroids improves chance of complete recovery; antiviral

NURSING MANAGEMENT: TAKE ACTION

1. Protect eye—use artificial tears; cover or patch at night.
   - Wear dark sunglasses.
   - Teach to report eye pain, drainage or discharge.
2. Encourage use of moist heat, facial massage to maintain muscle tone.
3. Teach to chew food on unaffected side.
4. Teach that the condition is usually self-limiting with minimal, if any, residual effects.
5. Provide support especially regarding physical appearance, which can be dramatic and devastating.

MIGRAINE HEADACHE SYMPTOMS

POUND

- **P**ulsating
- duration 4–72 h**O**urs
- **U**nilateral
- **N**ausea
- **D**isabling

May be preceded by an aura.

What You Need to Know
Migraine Headache Symptoms (POUND)

DEFINITION

Headache is a common symptom of various underlying pathologic conditions. With a migraine headache intracranial vessels spasm in response to a trigger. It is a recurrent headache disorder manifesting in attacks lasting 4 to 72 hours.

RISK FACTORS

- Female (menstrual cycle)
- Sleep pattern disruption
- Diet: skipped meals, red wine, chocolate, monosodium glutamate

RECOGNIZE AND ANALYZE CUES

- Intense, throbbing pain that may begin in the eye area
- May or may not have aura and visual disturbances
- Nausea, vomiting, photophobia
- Migraines can be seriously debilitating

MEDICAL MANAGEMENT: GENERATE SOLUTIONS

- Drugs: sumatriptan; dihydroergotamine mesylate, NSAIDs, aspirin, caffeine
  - Triptans work best when taken at the start of the headache; may be used for preventive treatment.
- Relaxation, yoga, stress management

NURSING MANAGEMENT: TAKE ACTION

1. Encourage to keep a headache diary to identify type of headache, triggers, etc.
2. Teach about lifestyle modifications and trigger identification.
   - Encourage consistent sleep hours and regular, well-balanced meals.
   - Promote ways to alleviate stress—relaxation, yoga, biofeedback.
3. Suggest cold compresses to area of pain; darkening the room (pulling down shades or closing curtains).
4. If patient falls asleep, allow them to remain undisturbed until they awaken.

Important nursing interventions	Serious/life-threatening implications
Common signs & symptoms	Patient teaching

TETANUS
(Lockjaw)

* Intact Sensorium

* Headache

* Difficulty Swallowing

* Irritability

* Tonic Spasms
  Leading to
  Laryngospasm

* Prevention—
  Childhood
  Immunizations

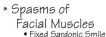

* Spasms of
  Facial Muscles
  • Fixed Sardonic Smile
  • Elevated Eyebrows

* Jaw Stiffness

* Fever

* Restlessness

* Exaggerated
  Reflexes

* Sweating

* Progressive
  Involvement Causes
  Opisthotonos

What You Need to Know
Tetanus

DEFINITION

Tetanus (lockjaw) is a severe nervous system infection affecting spinal and cranial nerves and is characterized by muscle rigidity and spasms due to production of a neurotoxin in infected wounds by *Clostridium tetani*, an anaerobic spore-forming gram-positive bacillus.

RISK FACTORS

- Inadequate immunization, injection drug use
- Chronic wounds, acute traumatic injury (exposure to soil or manure)

COMPLICATIONS

- Respiratory failure, fatal laryngospasm
- Severe tetanic muscle contractions → rhabdomyolysis, hyperkalemia, vertebral body and other fractures, muscle hemorrhages

RECOGNIZE AND ANALYZE CUES

- Progressive stiffness and tenderness in the muscles of the neck and jaw (trismus or lockjaw)
- Spasm of facial muscles produces "sardonic smile"
- Progressive involvement of trunk muscles → opisthotonos positioning
- Paroxysmal muscular contractions occur in response to stimuli (noise, touch, light)
- Remains alert; mental status not affected

MEDICAL MANAGEMENT: GENERATE SOLUTIONS

- Drugs: tetanus immune globulin to neutralize neurotoxin; tetanus toxoid on opposite arm, diazepam, vecuronium, antibiotics

NURSING MANAGEMENT: TAKE ACTION

1. Prevent tetanus by cleaning all wounds with soap and water and removing any foreign bodies.
   - Provide postexposure prophylaxis—tetanus toxoid (if previously immunized with three doses of DtaP, Tdap, or Td and it has been ≥10 years since the last dose).
2. Keep in a quiet, darkened room with minimum stimulus.
3. Monitor cardiac and respiratory status closely.
4. Be prepared to perform a tracheotomy to prevent fatal laryngospasm.

FRACTURE CLASSIFICATIONS

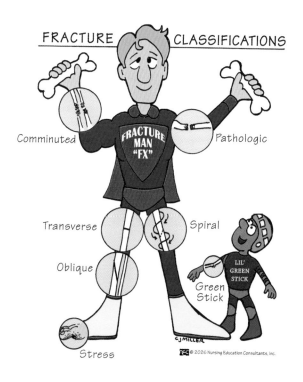

Comminuted

Pathologic

FRACTURE MAN "FX"

Transverse

Spiral

Oblique

Green Stick

LIL' GREEN STICK

Stress

CJ MILLER

Fracture Classification

DEFINITION
A fracture is a disruption or break in the bone and is classified by the direction of the fracture line in the bone.

RISK FACTORS
- Traumatic injuries
- Osteoporosis and cancer

COMPLICATIONS
- Refracture, nonunion, delayed union, or malunion
- Compartment syndrome—monitor fracture site for neurovascular changes (color, movement, sensation)
- Osteomyelitis

RECOGNIZE AND ANALYZE CUES
- Signs and symptoms: review figure
- Diagnostic: x-ray, CT scan, MRI

MEDICAL MANAGEMENT: GENERATE SOLUTIONS
- Cast application or splinting to immobilize fracture
- Closed reduction—nonsurgical; manual manipulation of fracture to realign bone
- Open reduction—surgery to realign bone
- External fixation—pins directly placed through the bone and secured in place by an external device
- Internal fixation—surgical incision is made and hardware (e.g., pins, rods, plates, etc.) is placed directly in the bone
- Skeletal traction—wire or metal pin is inserted directly into the bone
- Skin traction—noninvasive; force of pull applied to skin and indirectly to the bone

NURSING MANAGEMENT: TAKE ACTION
1. Assess neurovascular status of fractured extremity:
   - Immediately report unrelieved pain, paresthesia, absent pulses, swelling, pallor.
   - Administer prescribed analgesics.
2. Monitor cast during drying for denting or flattening.
   - Keep cast extremity elevated and apply ice packs (ensure cast stays dry) during first 24 hours after the cast application.
3. Assess surgical incision or pin sites for evidence of infection.
4. Teach patient about cast care or traction and measures to prevent complications.
5. Teach patient how to use assistive devices (e.g., walker, cane, crutches).

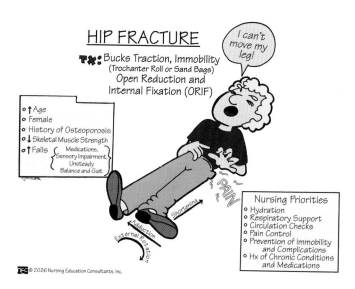

HIP FRACTURE

TX: Bucks Traction, Immobility
(Trochanter Roll or Sand Bags)
Open Reduction and
Internal Fixation (ORIF)

I can't move my leg!

- ↑ Age
- Female
- History of Osteoporosis
- ↓ Skeletal Muscle Strength
- ↑ Falls { Medications, Sensory Impairment, Unsteady Balance and Gait }

PAIN

Shortening

Adduction

External Rotation

Nursing Priorities
- Hydration
- Respiratory Support
- Circulation Checks
- Pain Control
- Prevention of Immobility and Complications
- Hx of Chronic Conditions and Medications

—— **What You Need to Know** ——

Hip Fracture

DEFINITION

The fracture involves the proximal third of the femur, which extends up to 5 cm below the lesser trochanter.

RISK FACTORS

- Female + age (prevalence greatest in females 65 years of age and older due to osteoporosis)
- Balance and gait problems
- Decreased skeletal strength
- Sensory impairment (vision/hearing)
- Medications
- Orthostatic hypotension

COMPLICATIONS

- Neurovascular compromise
- Infection; avascular necrosis
- Thromboembolism

RECOGNIZE AND ANALYZE CUES

- External rotation and adduction of the affected extremity
- Leg length shortening of affected extremity
- Severe pain, muscle spasms, tenderness

MEDICAL MANAGEMENT: GENERATE SOLUTIONS

- Initially, Buck's traction to immobilize fracture and decrease muscle spasms
- Surgical repair as soon as client's condition allows (permits earlier mobility and prevents complications of immobility)

NURSING MANAGEMENT: TAKE ACTION

1. Neurovascular checks distal to area of injury.
2. Position to prevent flexion, adduction, and internal rotation, which cause dislocation of the prosthesis.
3. Maintain affected leg in abducted position by placing abduction pillow between the legs.
4. Assess operative site for signs of bleeding.
5. Teach safety measures to prevent falls or hip dislocation after surgery.
   - Weight-bearing activities as prescribed
   - Use an elevated toilet seat
   - Maintain hip in neutral position

CARE OF PATIENT IN TRACTION

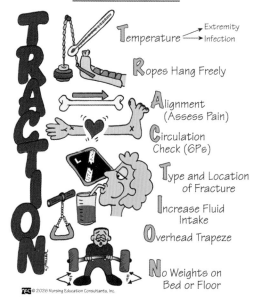

Temperature → Extremity
→ Infection

Ropes Hang Freely

Alignment (Assess Pain)

Circulation Check (6Ps)

Type and Location of Fracture

Increase Fluid Intake

Overhead Trapeze

No Weights on Bed or Floor

© 2026 Nursing Education Consultants, Inc.

What You Need to Know
Care of Patient in Traction

DEFINITION

Traction refers to the practice of slowly and gently pulling on a fractured or dislocated body part to decrease muscle spasm and reduce pain. Although not frequently used today, the two major types of traction are skin and skeletal traction.

TYPES OF TRACTION

- Skin traction involves the use of a Velcro boot (Buck's traction), belt, or halter, which is usually secured around the affected leg; weights are limited to 5 to 10 lb to prevent skin injury.
- Skeletal traction involves screws being surgically inserted directly into bone (e.g., femoral condyles for distal femur fractures), which allow the use of longer traction time and heavier weights (15–30 lb).

NURSING IMPLICATIONS: TAKE ACTION

1. Carefully assess for skin breakdown, especially underneath the affected extremity at least every 8 hours.
   - When possible, remove boot that is used for skin traction every 8 hours to inspect under the device and provide skin care.
2. Perform neurovascular checks on the extremity.
3. Do not change or remove traction weight on a client with continuous traction.
4. The traction ropes and weights should hang free from any obstructions.
5. Traction applied in one direction requires an equal countertraction to be effective.
6. Do not let the patient's feet touch the end of the bed; this will cause the countertraction to be lost.
7. Do not allow the traction weights to rest on anything at the end of the bed; this negates the pull of the traction.
8. Carefully assess the pin sites in clients with skeletal traction because osteomyelitis is a serious complication of skeletal traction.
9. An overhead trapeze bar can help the patient move up in the bed.

Important nursing interventions	Serious/life-threatening implications
Common signs & symptoms	Patient teaching

OSTEOARTHRITIS

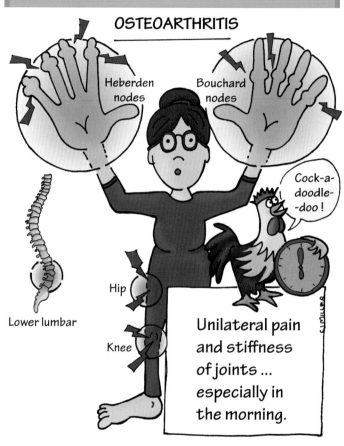

Osteoarthritis

DEFINITION

Osteoarthritis is a progressive, noninflammatory disease that causes a progressive degeneration of synovial joints. The cartilage at the ends of the long bones and in the intervertebral joints of the spine deteriorates and leaves the ends of the bones or vertebrae rubbing together; this produces a painful, swollen joint or spine.

RISK FACTORS

- Excessive use of a specific joint: knees in athletes, feet in dancers, etc.
- In males, hip is commonly affected; in females, hands are more commonly affected
- Obesity: joints that carry excess weight are more likely to degenerate earlier
- Older adults, especially females

COMPLICATIONS

- Neurovascular compromise
- Infection; avascular necrosis
- Thromboembolism

RECOGNIZE AND ANALYZE CUES

- Affects joints on one side of the body
- Involves weight-bearing joints; occurs because of mechanical stress
- May also involve joints in the fingers and the vertebral column
- Pain, swelling, tenderness, morning stiffness, instability
- Crepitation: a grating sound or feeling with movement
- Increased pain with activity
- Heberden nodes

MEDICAL MANAGEMENT

- Medications for pain relief: salicylates (aspirin), acetaminophen, NSAIDs (ibuprofen), COX-2 inhibitors (celecoxib)
- Intraarticular injection of corticosteroids
- Activity balanced with adequate rest
- Weight reduction, if appropriate
- Physical therapy and surgical intervention with joint replacement

NURSING IMPLICATIONS: TAKE ACTION

1. Acutely inflamed joints should be immobilized with splint or brace.
2. Plan ADLs to prevent stress on involved joints and provide adequate rest periods.
3. Heat compresses for relief of pain; cold compresses may be used if the joint is inflamed.
4. Teach to maintain a regular exercise program; decrease activity in acutely inflamed, painful joints.

RHEUMATOID ARTHRITIS

Boutonniere Deformity

Bilateral Ulnar Drift ("zig-zag Deformity")

Swan Neck Deformity

- Bilateral, symmetric joint involvement
- Commonly affects joints of hands and fingers
- Joint stiffness, pain, limitation of movement
- Joints are tender, painful, warm to the touch
- Joint pain increases with motion
- Morning stiffness lasting >1 hour
- Extraarticular Symptoms
  ◊ Rheumatoid nodules (located on bony areas exposed to pressure—fingers and elbows)
  ◊ Sjögren syndrome (decreased tearing, dry mouth, photosensitivity)

Hallux Valgas

─────── **What You Need to Know** ───────
Rheumatoid Arthritis

DEFINITION
Rheumatoid arthritis is a chronic, progressive, systemic inflammatory disease associated with severe morbidity and functional decline caused by inflammation of connective tissue, primarily in the synovial joints.

RISK FACTORS
- Sex: significantly increased incidence in females
- May occur at any age including childhood; peak incidence occurs between 30 and 60 years of age
- Genetic predisposition
- Occurs in all ethnic groups

RECOGNIZE AND ANALYZE CUES
- Bilateral, symmetric joint involvement (hands and feet)
- Swollen, warm, tender, red, painful joints; primarily affects small joints, wrists, elbows, shoulders
- Decrease in ROM, rheumatoid nodules over bony prominences
- Stiffness and pain are worse in the morning and decrease during the day with moderate activity.

MEDICAL MANAGEMENT
- Drug therapy: NSAIDs, corticosteroids for acute, severe exacerbations, methotrexate, disease-modifying antirheumatic drugs, and biologic response modifiers
- Heat and/or cold applications
- Rest and avoidance of repetitive movements
- Assistive devices and splints to preserve joints and prevent deformity
- Surgery: joint replacement
- Physical and rehabilitative therapy

NURSING IMPLICATIONS: TAKE ACTION
1. Teach about disease process, prescribed drug therapy.
2. Splint inflamed joints; provide assistance with ROM of affected joints.
3. Assist with self-care needs (bathing, feeding).
4. Avoid positions that precipitate joint contraction (sitting too long with knees bent).
5. Assist with identifying community resources.
6. Identify measures to assist in maintaining self-esteem: What activities can the patient continue to participate in? Focus on what the patient *can* do.

Important nursing interventions	Serious/life-threatening implications
Common signs & symptoms	Patient teaching

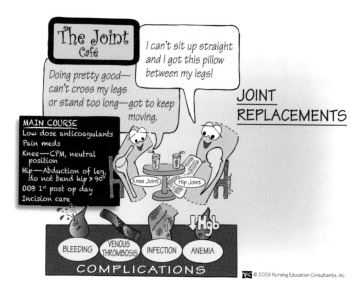

===== **What You Need to Know** =====

Joint Replacements

DEFINITION

A total joint arthroplasty is the surgical creation of a functional (synovial) joint using implants and is also known as total joint replacement. It is used most often to manage the pain of osteoarthritis and improve mobility.

COMPLICATIONS

- Infection, bleeding, anemia
- Venous thromboembolism (VTE)

NURSING IMPLICATIONS: TAKE ACTION

1. Preoperative care.
   - Teach the need to bathe with chlorhexidine gluconate (CHG) solution or wipes for at least the night before and the morning of surgery, as prescribed.
   - Teach the importance of sleeping on clean linens and not to use lotions or powders after the CHG baths; remind to avoid sleeping with pets in the bed.
   - Obtain an elevated toilet set; hip/knee replacement kit (utensils to assist with moving dressing, etc.).
2. Postoperative care: *total hip replacement*.
   - Position supine with the head slightly elevated, maintain abduction of the affected leg.
   - Monitor pain intensity and give prescribed analgesics.
   - Encourage quadriceps exercises, ankle pumps (pointing and flexing feet).
   - Legs should not be crossed (avoid adduction and internal rotation can lead to hip dislocation).
   - Perform neurovascular checks; monitor suture line.
   - Encourage mobility; may use antiembolism stockings and/or sequential compression devices to prevent venous stasis.
     - Cemented implant is usually allowed for immediate weight bearing.
     - Walker is used initially for stability and safety.
   - Administer anticoagulant drug therapy (usually low-dose aspirin) for 14 to 30 days following surgery to prevent VTE.
3. Postoperative care: *total knee replacement*
   - May have a knee compression dressing and immobilizer to keep the knee in extension.
   - Administer multimodal pain management.
   - Exercises: isometric quadriceps setting → straight-leg raises → gentle ROM → 90-degree knee flexion.

Important nursing interventions	Serious/life-threatening implications
Common signs & symptoms	Patient teaching

OSTEOPOROSIS RISK FACTORS

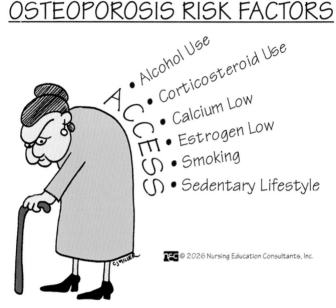

- A • Alcohol Use
- C • Corticosteroid Use
- C • Calcium Low
- E • Estrogen Low
- S • Smoking
- S • Sedentary Lifestyle

"Access" (leads to) Osteoporosis

What You Need to Know
Osteoporosis Risk Factors

DEFINITION

Osteoporosis is a chronic, progressive metabolic bone disease that involves an imbalance between new bone formation and bone resorption, which contributes to bone fragility.

RISK FACTORS

- Caucasian or Asian ethnicity, female sex, low body weight, small frame, and family history predisposes the person to decreased bone mineral density.
- Decreased intake of calcium and vitamin D delays bone remodeling.
- A sedentary lifestyle and a lack of weight-bearing activities increase bone resorption.
- Alcohol, smoking, lack of sunlight exposure, and caffeine slow down osteogenesis (new bone formation).
- Estrogen and testosterone inhibit bone loss; this is why advanced age and menopause are risk factors associated with this disease.
- Corticosteroids, thyroid hormones, heparin, long-acting sedatives, and antiseizure drugs interfere with calcium absorption and metabolism; this leads to decreased bone mineral density.

RECOGNIZE AND ANALYZE CUES

- History of fractures; asymptomatic before fracture
- Back pain
- Decreased mobility
- Dowager hump—kyphosis of spine
- Loss of height by several inches—due to vertebral fractures
- Diagnosis is made by dual-energy x-ray absorptiometry (DEXA) scan—provides bone mineral density (BMD) of the spine and hip.
  - When the BMD is less than 2.5 standard deviations below the mean BMD of young adults, osteoporosis is confirmed; reported as a T-score less than or equal to -2.5 (the greater the negative number, the more severe the osteoporosis).
  - DEXA scan is recommended for all females over the age of 65 years, postmenopausal over 50, and for everyone with a suspected osteoporotic fracture.

OSTEOPOROSIS
(After Menopause—↓Estrogen)

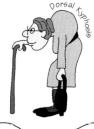

Dorsal Kyphosis

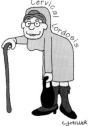

Cervical Lordosis

C.J.MILLER

Generalized progressive reduction of bone density, causing weakness of skeletal strength.

Slender, Female, Caucasian, Alcohol Users, Smokers, Steroid Users, Inactive Lifestyles, and Diets Low in Calcium or Vitamin D Deficiency... have the highest risk.

Fractures especially at T-8 & below... Hip & Colles' fractures most common.

What You Need to Know
Osteoporosis

MEDICAL MANAGEMENT

- Dietary: increased intake of protein, calcium, and vitamin D.
- Calcium supplements: daily intake of calcium should be approximately 1000 mg for males and postmenopausal females between the ages of 50 and 70 years and 1200 mg for those over the age of 70.
- Vitamin D supplements: (800–1000 IU recommended daily for males and postmenopausal females over the age of 50 years) to enhance the utilization of calcium; spending 20 minutes daily in the sun will provide adequate vitamin D.
- Antiresorptive medications, such as bisphosphonates and calcitonin, facilitate increased bone density.
- Weight-bearing exercise: activities that put moderate stress on bones by working them against gravity (e.g., walking, racquet sports, jogging).

NURSING IMPLICATIONS: TAKE ACTION

1. Assess patient's pain and administer prescribed medications. Hot/cold therapy, short periods of rest, and a firm mattress may also reduce pain.
2. Patients taking bisphosphonates should be instructed to take the medication 30 minutes before meals with a full glass of water and to sit upright for 30 minutes after taking to prevent esophageal irritation.
3. Advise patient taking calcium supplements to divide doses to increase calcium absorption.
4. Consult with dietitian about food sources high in calcium (e.g., dairy products, almonds, sardines, salmon).
5. Teach body mechanics—avoid twisting motions, prolonged bending, and standing.
6. Encourage outdoor physical activity for 30 minutes daily to get more vitamin D, strengthen muscles, and improve balance.

Important nursing interventions   Serious/life-threatening implications

Common signs & symptoms   Patient teaching

NURSING CARE FOR SPRAINS AND STRAINS

R Rest
I Ice
C Compression
E Elevation

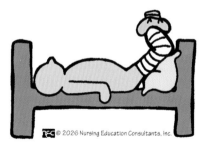

What You Need to Know
Sprains and Strains—Nursing Care

DEFINITION

Sprains—Injury to ligaments and supporting muscle fiber surrounding a joint. Classified by the degree of ligament damage (first [mild], second [moderate], and third degree [severe]). *Strains*—Pulled muscle injury (may involve tendon). Classified as first degree (mild or slightly pulled muscle), second degree (moderate or moderately torn muscle), and third degree (severe muscle tear or muscle rupture).

RISK FACTORS

- Trauma
- Repetitive use
- Overuse
- Inadequate rest during exercise or activity
- Athletes

RECOGNIZE AND ANALYZE CUES

- Pain, swelling, redness at injured site
- Decreased mobility of affected extremity and bruising
- Muscle spasms, neurovascular changes (skin color, mobility, sensation)
- Common sites of sprains: wrist, knee, ankle
- Common sites of strains: lower back, hamstrings, calf

MEDICAL MANAGEMENT

- Diagnostics: x-rays can determine whether a fracture has occurred; MRI may be ordered to identify a muscle, tendon, or ligament tear
- Give tetanus prophylaxis and antibiotics for open fractures
- Analgesics for pain management
- Surgical repair may be done for severe injury to ligament

NURSING IMPLICATIONS: TAKE ACTION

1. Assess for changes in neurovascular status: pulse, temperature, capillary refill, and movement of affected extremity
2. Elevate affected extremity above heart level and apply compression bandage. Ice packs of injury for 15 to 30 at a time for 2 to 3 days.
3. After acute phase; 24 to 48 hours, recommend that moist heat be applied to the affected area, not to exceed 20 to 30 minutes.
4. Consult with physical therapy and teach patient exercises that improve muscle strength and function.
5. Educate the patient on taking measures (warm-up prior to exercise, stretch after exercise) to prevent reinjury.

MENOPAUSE

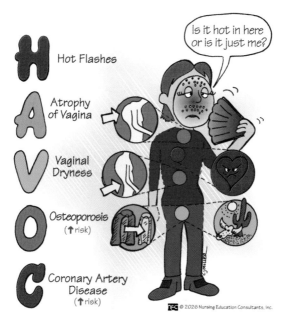

What You Need to Know
Menopause

DEFINITION

Menopause is the ceasing of menses for 12 consecutive months and usually occurs between the ages of 40 and 58 with a mean age of 51 years. Perimenopause is the period that encompasses the transition from normal ovulatory cycles to the cessation of menses and is characterized by irregular menstrual cycles. Climacteric is the period when a female moves from the reproductive stage of life through the perimenopausal transition and menopause to the postmenopausal years.

RISK FACTORS

- Aging
- Surgical menopause—removal of ovaries
- Primary ovarian insufficiency—irregularity or cessation of ovulatory cycles before age 40 years

COMPLICATIONS

- Osteoporosis
- Coronary artery disease

RECOGNIZE AND ANALYZE CUES

- Perimenopausal—irregular cycles with heavy bleeding following by ↓bleeding
- Vasomotor symptoms (hot flashes or flushes)—sudden warm sensations, visible red flush to skin, perspiration, night sweats
- Genitourinary—vaginal dryness, urinary incontinence, recurrent urinary tract infection, dyspareunia, uterine prolapse
- Mood and behavioral changes—anxiety, depressed mood, insomnia (related to hot flashes and night sweats)

MEDICAL MANAGEMENT: GENERATE SOLUTIONS

- Drugs: menopausal hormone therapy; selective serotonin reuptake inhibitors (SSRIs), serotonin-norepinephrine reuptake inhibitors (SNRIs), gabapentin, clonidine, oxybutynin to ↓hot flashes; vaginal creams, lubricants for vaginal dryness and atrophy
- Alternative therapies: homeopathy, acupuncture, herbs, yoga

NURSING MANAGEMENT: TAKE ACTION

1. Teach to wear layered clothing and avoid triggers for hot flashes (heat, stress, caffeine, alcohol, tobacco, spicy foods).
2. Encourage a calcium-rich diet and vitamin D supplementation.
3. Encourage regular exercise >30 minutes, three times weekly.
4. Teach about hormone therapy.

POST-MASTECTOMY
NURSING CARE

- Elevate affected side with distal joint higher than proximal joint.

- No BP, injections or venipunctures on affected side.

- Watch for S & S of edema on affected arm.
  (edema may occur post op or years later)

- Lymphedema can occur any time after
  axillary node disection.

- Flexion and extension exercises of the hand in recovery.

- Abduction and external rotation arm exercises
  after wound has healed.

- Assess dressing for drainage.

- Assess wound drain for amount and color.

- Provide privacy when patient looks at incision.

- Chemotherapy, Radiation therapy.

- Monitor for Complications — hemorrhage, hematoma,
  lymphedema, infection, post-mastectomy pain syndrome.

- Psychological concerns:
  Altered body image
  Altered sexuality
  Fear of disease outcome

Reproductive

What You Need to Know
Post-Mastectomy Nursing Care

DEFINITION

Breast cancer is the most commonly diagnosed cancer among females.

RISK FACTORS

- Family history, genetic factors (mutation of BRCA1 or BRCA2 genes and others)
- Age ≥55 years, radiation exposure, chemicals in environment
- Sedentary lifestyle, smoking, ↑ fat intake, obesity, nightshift work, alcohol use

COMPLICATIONS

- Recurrence
- Metastasis to bone, liver, lung, brain

RECOGNIZE AND ANALYZE CUES

- Lump or thickening in the upper, outer quadrant of the breast; usually painless
- Nipple discharge (maybe bloody) or retraction
- Peau d'orange appearance (dimpling, edema, pitting of skin)
- Diagnosis: mammogram, biopsy, axillary lymph node analysis

MEDICAL MANAGEMENT: GENERATE SOLUTIONS

- Surgery: lumpectomy or mastectomy; reconstructive surgery
- Radiation: external radiation, brachytherapy, palliative radiation therapy
- Drugs: chemotherapy, hormone therapy, immunotherapy, targeted therapy

NURSING MANAGEMENT: TAKE ACTION

1. Review figure for post-mastectomy nursing care for the first 24 to 48 hours.
2. Anticipate the patient will be discharged early, if no postoperative problems.
3. Teach about additional post-mastectomy strengthening arm exercises as prescribed—hand wall climbing, rope turning, side bends, shoulder blade squeeze.

Important nursing interventions	Serious/life-threatening implications
Common signs & symptoms	Patient teaching

TURP

(Transurethral Resection of the Prostate)

- Continuous or Intermittent Bladder Irrigation (C.B.I.)
  (Usually DC'd after 24 hours, if No Clots). Murphy Drip

- Close observation of drainage system-
  (↑Bladder Distention causes Pain & Bleeding).

- Maintain Catheter Patency

- Bladder Spasms

- Pain Control: Analgesics & ↓Activity first 24 hours.

- Avoid straining with BMs. ↑Fiber diet & Laxatives.

- Complications:
  - Hemorrhage—Bleeding should gradually ↓
    to light pink in 24 hours.
  - Urinary Incontinence—Kegel Exercises
  - Infections—↑Fluids
  - Prevent deep vein thrombosis
  - Sequential compression stockings
  - Discourage sitting for prolonged periods

What You Need to Know
TURP

DEFINITION

Transurethral resection of the prostate (TURP) involves removal of prostate tissue using a resectoscope inserted through the urethra. TURP is a closed surgical procedure and is the gold standard for the treatment of obstructing benign prostatic hyperplasia (BPH).

RISK FACTORS FOR BPH

- Increasing age, obesity (↑ waist circumference)
- Lack of physical activity, ↑ intake of red meat and animal fat
- Alcohol use, erectile dysfunction, smoking, diabetes
- Family history (first-degree relative)

POSTOPERATIVE COMPLICATIONS

- Hemorrhage, bladder spasms
- Urinary incontinence, infection

RECOGNIZE AND ANALYZE CUES FOR BPH

- Nocturia, urinary hesitancy, frequency, urgency, dribbling
- Decrease in force of urinary stream, sensation of incomplete emptying of the bladder
- Urinary retention may cause overflow urinary incontinence and dribbling after voiding
- Diagnostics: digital rectal exam, transrectal ultrasound, urinalysis with culture and sensitivity, MRI, prostate-specific antigen blood test to rule out cancer

MEDICAL MANAGEMENT: GENERATE SOLUTIONS

- Drugs: 5α-reductase inhibitors (finasteride, dutasteride), α-adrenergic receptor blockers (doxazosin, tamsulosin), and combination drugs from the two categories
- Complementary health (herbal therapy): saw palmetto

NURSING MANAGEMENT: TAKE ACTION

1. Provide preoperative care.
   - Administer antibiotics.
   - Insert a urinary catheter, if prescribed, to restore bladder drainage.
2. Provide postoperative care—review figure.
3. Provide discharge instructions on how to care for the urinary catheter, manage urinary incontinence while bladder heals, report signs of infection, prevent constipation, avoid heavy lifting, refrain from intercourse, and driving as directed by healthcare provider.

Important nursing interventions

Common signs & symptoms

Serious/life-threatening implications

Patient teaching

URINARY TRACT INFECTION (UTI)

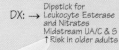

CYSTITIS:
Frequency
Urgency
Suprapubic Pain
Dysuria
Hematuria
Fever
Confusion
in Older Adults

PYELONEPHRITIS:
Flank Pain
Dysuria
Mild Fatigue, Malaise
Chills, Fever, Vomiting
Pain at Costovertebral
Angle
Same S & S as Cystitis

DX: → Dipstick for Leukocyte Esterase and Nitrates
Midstream UA/C & S
↑ Risk in older adults

TX: → Antibiotics
↑ Fluid Intake
Prevention

NURSING GOALS:
Cystitis
• Symptomatic Relief
• Teaching & Prevention
• Showers Better Than Baths
• Perineal Cleansing "Front To Back"
• Voiding After Intercourse
• Antimicrobial Therapy
• No Scented Toilet Paper
• No Perfumes, Etc. to Perineal Area
• Empty Bladder Regularly
Pyelonephritis
• May Require Hospitalization
• Severe Cases–IV Antibiotics Initially
• Monitor for Urosepsis to Prevent Septic Shock

© 2026 Nursing Education Consultants, Inc.

What You Need to Know
Urinary Tract Infection (UTI)

DEFINITION

Urinary tract infection (UTI) is the presence of microorganisms within the urinary tract causing an infection. *Escherichia coli* is the most common microorganism causing a UTI.

RISK FACTORS

- Female adult urethra is short with close proximity to rectum and vagina
- Diabetes, aging, HIV infection
- Urinary obstruction and stasis—tumors, renal calculi, neurogenic bladder
- Foreign bodies—urinary catheters, cystoscopy
- Poor hygiene, intercourse (female)

COMPLICATIONS

- Lower UTI may progress to an upper UTI
- Urosepsis, chronic pyelonephritis

RECOGNIZE AND ANALYZE CUES

- Review figure for symptoms of lower UTI (cystitis) and upper UTI (pyelonephritis) and diagnostic test
- Upper UTI has systemic symptoms; lower UTI does not usually have systemic symptoms
- Symptoms of UTI are different in older adults with abdominal discomfort instead of dysuria and suprapubic pain and cognitive impairment (e.g., confusion)

MEDICAL MANAGEMENT: GENERATE SOLUTIONS

- Drugs: antibiotics (trimethoprim/sulfamethoxazole, nitrofurantoin, fosfomycin, cephalexin); urinary analgesic (phenazopyridine)

NURSING MANAGEMENT: TAKE ACTION

1. Teach importance of taking all doses of antibiotics, emptying the bladder regularly and completely, wiping from front to back (females), drinking at least 2 to 3 L/day, voiding before and after intercourse.
2. Prevent catheter-associated urinary tract infections (CAUTIs).
   - Avoid unnecessary catheterization; early removal of indwelling catheters.

URINARY CALCULI

- ↑ Incidence in Males

- Nausea & Vomiting

- Agonizing Flank Pain
  May Radiate To:
    Groin
    Testicles
    Abdominal Area

- Sharp, Sudden,
  Severe Pain:
  (May be intermittent
  depending on
  stone movement)

- Hematuria

- Dysuria

- Urinary Frequency

- Diagnosis
  Ultrasound, CT Scan
  Intravenous pyelogram (IVP)
  Kidney Stone Analysis
  Retrograde pyelogram
  Cystoscopy
  Measure Urine pH

- Risk Factors - Etiology
  Infection
  Urinary Stasis & Retention
  Immobility, Sedentary Occupation
  Dehydration, Warm Climates
  ↑Uric Acid (Gout)
  ↑Urinary Oxalate
  Obesity, Diabetes
  Family History

What You Need to Know
Urinary Calculi

DEFINITION

Urolithiasis is stone (calculus) formation within the urinary tract. Stones (calculi) usually do not cause symptoms until they move into the lower urinary tract, then they can cause severe pain.

RISK FACTORS

- Review figure

COMPLICATIONS

- Urinary obstruction, injury to urinary tract, kidney failure
- Recurrent stone formation, sepsis

RECOGNIZE AND ANALYZE CUES

- Review figure for signs and symptoms
- Types of urinary calculi:
  - Calcium oxalate: most common type; ↑males, tend to be small; account for 70% to 80% of all upper urinary tract calculi
  - Calcium phosphate: typically a mixed stone with struvite or oxalate
  - Struvite: contain bacteria and tend to be large; large staghorn type; ↑females
  - Uric acid: occur most often with primary or secondary problems of uric acid metabolism (gout); ↑males
  - Cystine: autosomal recessive defect; defective absorption of cystine in GI and kidney, causing excess concentration leading to stone formation

MEDICAL MANAGEMENT: GENERATE SOLUTIONS

- Drugs: opioid analgesics, thiazide diuretics (calcium oxalate), allopurinol (uric acid), antibiotics (struvite), potassium citrate (cystine)
- Lithotripsy: outpatient procedure; delivers sound or shock waves to break up stone
- Surgery: percutaneous ureterolithotomy, pyelolithotomy, or nephrolithotomy

NURSING MANAGEMENT: TAKE ACTION

1. Administer medications as prescribed for pain, etc.
2. Strain urine to monitor passage of stone.
3. Teach about general prevention—maintaining adequate hydration, ↓salt and meat intake, avoid oxalate rich food, other diet modifications.

ACUTE KIDNEY INJURY (AKI)

Risk—First Stage of AKI—Creatinine ↑ x 1.5 or GFR ↓ 25%
Urine Output <0.5 mL/kg/hr for 6 hours

Injury—Second Stage—Creatinine ↑ x 2 or GFR ↓ 50%
Urine Output <0.5 mL/kg/hr for 12 hours

Failure—Third Stage—Creatinine ↑ x 3
or GFR ↓ 75% or Creatinine > 4 mg/dL
Urine Output <0.3 mL/kg/hr for 24 hours
(oliguria) or Anuria for 12 hours

Loss—Fourth Stage—Persistent Acute
Kidney Failure; Loss of Function > 4 weeks

End-Stage Kidney Disease—Complete Loss
of Kidney Function > 3 months

Urinary—Kidney

What You Need to Know
Acute Kidney Injury (AKI)—Stages

DEFINITION

AKI is a clinical syndrome with abrupt loss of kidney function that may occur over several hours or days, and is characterized by uremia. The **RIFLE** classification describes the stages of AKI. RIFLE is an acronym of **R**isk, **I**njury, **F**ailure, **L**oss, **E**nd-stage kidney disease.

CAUSES

- Prerenal—reduce system circulation → ↓renal blood flow
  - ↓Cardiac output (heart failure [HF], myocardial infarction [MI], shock, dysrhythmias)
  - Hypovolemia (burns, dehydration, hemorrhage)
  - ↓Renal blood flow (renal artery stenosis/embolism
  - Anaphylaxis, septic shock, liver failure
- Intrarenal—result of kidney damage → ↓nephron function
  - Acute tubular necrosis (ATN)—from radiographic contrast material, aminoglycosides, NSAIDs, nephrotoxic substances
  - Acute interstitial nephritis, glomerulonephritis
  - Nephrotoxic injury—hemolytic transfusion reaction, crush injury
  - Systemic lupus erythematosus, thrombotic disorders, preeclampsia/eclampsia
- Postrenal—involves obstruction of urine flow → reflux of urine into renal pelvis → ↓kidney function
  - Benign prostatic hypertrophy; prostate, colon, or bladder cancer
  - Urinary calculi, neurogenic bladder, trauma (back, pelvis, perineum)

RECOGNIZE AND ANALYZE CUES

- Can develop over hours or days
- Potentially reversible; high mortality rate
- Review figure for stages of AKI, which describes serum creatinine, glomerular filtration rate (GFR), urine output

| Important nursing interventions | Serious/life-threatening implications |
| Common signs & symptoms | Patient teaching |

ACUTE KIDNEY INJURY (AKI)

- SIGNS and SYMPTOMS -

Oliguric Phase
- Oliguria—<400 mL/day; occurs within 1–7 days of kidney injury
- Urinalysis—casts, RBCs, WBCs, sp gr fixated at 1.010
- Metabolic Acidosis
- Hyperkalemia and Hyponatremia
- Elevated BUN and Creatinine
- Fatigue and Malaise

Diuretic Phase
- Gradual ↑ in urine output—1–3 L/day; may reach 3–5 L/day
- Hypovolemia, Dehydration, Hypotension
- Hyponatremia, Hypokalemia
- BUN and Creatinine Levels Begin to Normalize

Recovery Phase
- Begins when GFR Increases
- BUN and Creatinine Levels Plateau, then ↓

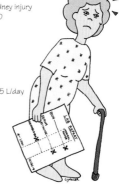

© 2026 Nursing Education Consultants, Inc.

What You Need to Know

Acute Kidney Injury (AKI)—Phases

DEFINITION

AKI progresses through three phases—oliguric, diuretic, and recovery. The stages provide a framework for understanding the signs and symptoms of AKI.

COMPLICATIONS

- Infection (leading cause of death)

RECOGNIZE AND ANALYZE CUES

- Oliguric phase
    - Lasts an average of 10 to 14 days; can last for months
    - Urine output can assist in determining the cause of AKI—anuria (urinary tract obstruction; postrenal cause); oliguria (prerenal cause); nonoliguric (ATN, acute interstitial nephritis; intrarenal)
    - May have proteinuria if glomerulus is affected
- Diuretic phase
    - May last 1 to 3 weeks
    - Acid-base balance, electrolytes, BUN, creatinine levels normalize
- Recovery phase
    - Improvements noted within the first 2 weeks
    - May take 12 months for kidney function to stabilize
    - May progress to end-stage renal disease
    - Older adult often does not have complete kidney recovery

MEDICAL MANAGEMENT: GENERATE SOLUTIONS

- Treat cause of AKI
- Drugs: diuretics, ↓potassium levels—sodium polystyrene sulfonate (kayexalate)
- Renal replacement therapy (RRT), peritoneal dialysis (not used often), intermittent hemodialysis, continuous RRT
- Nutrition: Intake of protein, potassium, and sodium is regulated according to serum plasma levels; ↑carbohydrate and fats; may need parenteral nutrition

NURSING MANAGEMENT: TAKE ACTION

1. Monitor vital signs, fluid/electrolyte balance, urine output.
2. Maintain nutrition; take daily weights.
3. Prevent infection.

Important nursing interventions	Serious/life-threatening implications
Common signs & symptoms	Patient teaching

CHRONIC KIDNEY DISEASE (CKD)

ESRD—END-STAGE KIDNEY DISEASE

↓ 15 mL/min GFR

- Neurologic
  Weakness/Fatigue
  Headache
  Sleep Disturbances

- Psychologic
  Withdrawn
  Behavior Changes
  Depression

- Cardiovascular
  ↑ BP
  Pitting Edema
  Periorbital Edema
  Heart Failure
  Pericarditis
  Peripheral Artery Disease

- Hematologic
  Anemia
  Bleeding Tendencies
  Infection

- Fld/Lytes— ↑ Potassium
  Acid/Base—Metabolic Acidosis

- Pulmonary
  Pulmonary Edema
  Uremic Pleuritis
  Pneumonia

- Skin
  Dry Flaky
  Pruritus
  Ecchymosis
  Yellow-Gray Skin Color

- GI
  Ammonia Odor to Breath
  Metallic Taste
  Mouth/Gum Ulcerations
  Anorexia
  Nausea/Vomiting
  GI Bleeding

- Musculoskeletal
  Cramps
  Renal Osteodystrophy
  Bone Pain

—Hemodialysis—
- Evaluate access site for patency & signs of infection.
- **DO NOT** take BP, insert IV line, or perform venipuncture in extremity with vascular access.

What You Need to Know
Chronic Kidney Disease (CKD)—End Stage

DEFINITION

CKD is a progressive, irreversible reduction in kidney function such that the kidneys are no longer able to maintain the body environment. The GFR gradually decreases as the nephrons are destroyed.

RISK FACTORS

- Chronic hypertension, diabetes
- Chronic glomerulonephritis, pyelonephritis
- Exposure to nephrotoxic drugs or chemicals
- Ethnic minority—↑Black Americans and Native Americans
- Autoimmune disease
- Age >60 years
- Family history of CKD

RECOGNIZE AND ANALYZE CUES

- GFR is the preferred way to determine kidney function rather than serum creatinine levels.
- Review figure.

MEDICAL MANAGEMENT: GENERATE SOLUTIONS

- Drugs: calcium supplementation, phosphate binders, antihypertensives (angiotensin-converting enzyme inhibitors or angiotensin receptor blockers), erythropoietin, antihyperlipidemics (statins), vitamins
- RRT: dialysis, kidney transplant

NURSING MANAGEMENT: TAKE ACTION

1. Monitor hydration status, identify signs of fluid and electrolyte imbalance (e.g., hypocalcemia, hyperkalemia), identify interventions to correct imbalances.
2. Encourage nutritional intake within dietary guidelines (sodium, potassium, phosphate, fluid restrictions).
3. Assess for bleeding tendencies; monitor laboratory results.
4. Monitor daily weight and report any weight gain >4 lb.
5. Provide support about lifestyle changes, living with a chronic illness, decisions about type of dialysis or transplantation.

POST–KIDNEY TRANSPLANT REJECTION SIGNS

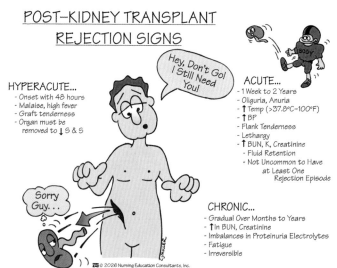

HYPERACUTE...
- Onset with 48 hours
- Malaise, high fever
- Graft tenderness
- Organ must be removed to ↓ S & S

ACUTE...
- 1 Week to 2 Years
- Oliguria, Anuria
- ↑ Temp (>37.8°C–100°F)
- ↑ BP
- Flank Tenderness
- Lethargy
- ↑ BUN, K, Creatinine
- Fluid Retention
- Not Uncommon to Have at Least One Rejection Episode

CHRONIC...
- Gradual Over Months to Years
- ↑ In BUN, Creatinine
- Imbalances in Proteinuria Electrolytes
- Fatigue
- Irreversible

© 2026 Nursing Education Consultants, Inc.

— What You Need to Know —
Kidney Transplant Rejection

DEFINITION

The transplantation of a kidney is from a compatible blood–typed deceased donor, blood relative, or live donor. The transplanted kidney is placed extraperitoneal in the iliac fossa (usually on the right side to facilitate anastomosis and decrease the occurrence of ileus), most commonly on the right lower side of the abdomen. *Rejection* is a major problem after a kidney transplant.

COMPLICATIONS OF KIDNEY TRANSPLANT

- Rejection, infection, cardiovascular disease, cancer
- Recurrence of kidney disease, corticosteroid-related problems

RECOGNIZE AND ANALYZE CUES

- Hyperacute—occurs quickly within 48 hours
- Acute—most common type; occurs within 1 week →2 years
- Chronic—occurs gradually over months to years

MEDICAL MANAGEMENT: GENERATE SOLUTIONS

- Drugs: immunosuppressants, corticosteroids
- Hyperacute: immediate surgical removal of transplanted kidney
- Acute: ↑dose of immunosuppressants
- Chronic: conservative management until dialysis is necessary

NURSING MANAGEMENT: TAKE ACTION

1. Monitor fluid and electrolyte balance; signs of infection.
2. Teach about immunosuppressive therapy.

Important nursing interventions	Serious/life-threatening implications
Common signs & symptoms	Patient teaching

URINARY DIVERSIONS

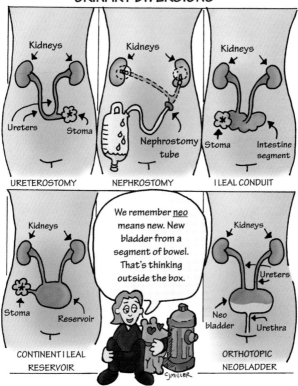

What You Need to Know
Urinary Diversion

DEFINITION
A urinary diversion is a means of diverting urinary output from the bladder to an external device or via a different path out of the body. There are incontinent urinary diversions, continent urinary diversions, and orthotopic bladder reconstruction or orthotopic neobladder.

RISK FACTORS
- Bladder cancer, neurogenic bladder, congenital anomalies
- Strictures, trauma to the bladder, chronic bladder inflammation

COMPLICATIONS
- Infection, obstruction

RECOGNIZE AND ANALYZE CUES
- Incontinent urinary diversions
    - Ureterostomy—ureter removed from bladder and brought through abdominal wall with the creation of a stoma; may be done to one or both kidneys or both ureters anastomosed together and brought up to one stoma
    - Nephrostomy—catheter inserted into kidney pelvis; may be done to one or both kidneys; may be temporary or permanent
    - Ileal conduit or loop—a piece of the ileum is used to create a pouch with both ureters sutured into the pouch and a stoma is created on the abdomen; urine cannot be stored, so an ostomy bag (appliance) is used to collect and hold urine
- Continent urinary diversions
    - Continent urinary reservoir—Kock, Indiana (most often used), Miami—created from a distal part of the ileum and proximal part of the colon; ureters are inserted into the reservoir; a surgically created valve prevents involuntary leakage; reservoir needs catheterized four to six times a day
    - Orthotopic neobladder—existing bladder is removed and an internal pouch is formed from part of the intestine; pouch is the neobladder that stores urine

NURSING MANAGEMENT: TAKE ACTION
1. Teach about care of the urinary diversion and monitoring for obstruction or infection.
2. Provide referral to ostomy nurse.

Important nursing interventions	Serious/life-threatening implications
Common signs & symptoms	Patient teaching

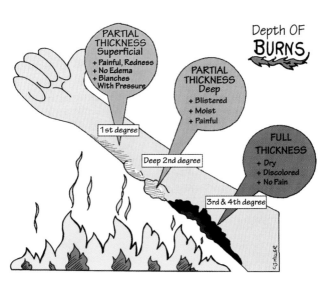

What You Need to Know
Depth of Burns

DEFINITION

Burns are tissue injuries caused by heat (thermal; the most common type of injury), cold (frostbite), chemical (acids, alkalines), inhalation, friction, electrical current, or radiation. The severity of a burn is classified by the depth of the burn, extent of the burn, location of the burn, preexisting health issues, and other related injuries.

BURN DEPTH CLASSIFICATION

- Four factors influence burn depth:
  - Temperature of burn agent
  - Duration of contact
  - Thickness of epidermis and dermis
  - Blood supply to burn area
- Partial-thickness
  - Superficial (involves epidermis; dry, pink to red color); 1st degree
  - Deep (involves epidermis and dermis; moist, red, blistered); 2nd degree
- Full-thickness
  - Damage to entire thickness of skin, local nerve endings destroyed
  - Appearance—3rd degree dry, waxy white, brown, leathery; 4th degree black, charred

EXTENT OF BURN

- Rule of Nines—used for initial triage assessment for adults
- Lund-Browder chart—used to assess burns in children
- More accurate assessment is completed in the burn unit to measure percentage of total body surface area (TBSA) burned

LOCATION OF BURN

- Location of burn directs treatment
  - Face, neck, chest areas → inhalation injury
  - Hand, foot, joint areas → ↓mobility and function
  - Buttocks, perineum → infection from urine, feces contamination
  - Circumferential burns → ↓blood supply distal to injury

RISK FACTORS

- History of diabetes or peripheral vascular disease → delayed healing (foot, leg burns)
- Preexisting chronic illness → poor prognosis because burn injury put ↑stress on body

---

| Important nursing interventions | Serious/life-threatening implications |
| Common signs & symptoms | Patient teaching |

LYME DISEASE

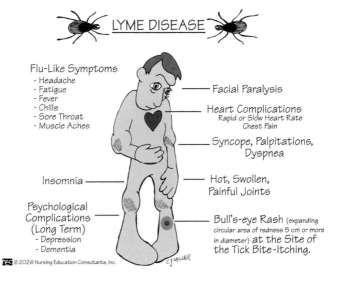

Flu-Like Symptoms
- Headache
- Fatigue
- Fever
- Chills
- Sore Throat
- Muscle Aches

— Facial Paralysis

— Heart Complications
Rapid or Slow Heart Rate
Chest Pain

— Syncope, Palpitations, Dyspnea

Insomnia —

— Hot, Swollen, Painful Joints

Psychological Complications (Long Term)
- Depression
- Dementia

— Bull's-eye Rash (expanding circular area of redness 5 cm or more in diameter) at the Site of the Tick Bite-Itching.

CJ MILLER

Integumentary

What You Need to Know
Lyme Disease

DEFINITION

Lyme disease is the most common vector-borne disease in the United States and is an inflammatory response to the spirochete (spiral-shaped bacteria) *Borrelia burgdorferi*. If not treated with antibiotics, complications of later disease occur.

RISK FACTORS

- Bite by an infected deer tick
- Residence or recreation in wooded areas of northeastern United States from Maine to Maryland and the upper midwestern states of Minnesota and Wisconsin

COMPLICATIONS

- Chronic arthritis pain, joint swelling, carditis
- Posttreatment Lyme disease syndrome: pain, fatigue, or difficulty thinking that last for >6 months after treatment is completed

RECOGNIZE AND ANALYZE CUES

- Erythema migrans (bull's eye rash)—a characteristic early symptom
- Diagnostics—serum enzyme immunoassay followed by immunoblot (western blot)

MEDICAL MANAGEMENT: GENERATE SOLUTIONS

- Drugs: antibiotics (doxycycline, cefuroxime, amoxicillin)

NURSING MANAGEMENT: TAKE ACTION

1. Teach to check for ticks often; avoid walking through tall grass or low brush or sitting on logs.
2. Teach to avoid heavily wooded areas; use insect repellent (DEET); wear long-sleeved tops and long pants and closed-toe shoes (when outdoors hiking); tuck pants into boots or long socks.
3. Teach to immediately remove any ticks with fine-tipped tweezers; remove by grasping tick as close to skin as possible and pulling straight out. Do not twist or jerk; never crush a tick with fingers. Wash bitten area with soap and water, iodine scrub, or rubbing alcohol; apply antiseptic.
4. Teach to avoid "painting" the tick with nail polish or petroleum jelly or using heat to detach ticks from skin.

MELANOMA
(SIGNS OF)

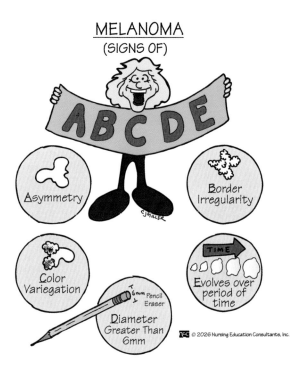

ABCDE

Asymmetry

Border Irregularity

Color Variegation

Diameter Greater Than 6mm

6mm Pencil Eraser

Evolves over period of time

TIME

What You Need to Know
Melanoma

DEFINITION

Melanoma is a type of skin cancer that arises from the melanocytes (cells that make melanin) and is characterized by a sudden or progressive change in size, symmetry, color, elevation, or shape of a mole. It is the leading cause of skin cancer deaths.

RISK FACTORS

- UV radiation, tanning bed use, high familial incidence
- Red or blond hair, blue- or light-colored eyes, light-colored skin that freckles easily

COMPLICATIONS

- Metastatic spread and subsequent death

RECOGNIZE AND ANALYZE CUES

- Change in a pigmented lesion: either hypo- or hyperpigmentation, bleeding, scaling, ulceration, or changes in size or texture
- Any new and/or changing nevus (mole)
- Most common sites in males are back, then chest; in females, legs and then back
- Diagnostics: dermoscopy (magnifies lesions), full-thickness excisional biopsy

MEDICAL MANAGEMENT: GENERATE SOLUTIONS

- Depends on site of tumor and stage of cancer
- Surgery: wide surgical excision, possible sentinel node biopsy
- Immunotherapy (cytokines, PD-1 inhibitors, CTLA-4 inhibitors); targeted therapy (BRAF and MEK inhibitors); chemotherapy and/or radiation therapy

NURSING MANAGEMENT: TAKE ACTION

1. Teach the importance of avoiding unnecessary exposure to sunlight; apply protective sunscreen when outside; wear a hat, opaque clothing, sunglasses when in the sun.
2. Teach the warning signs of skin cancer and to examine body once a month looking for skin changes and reporting any changes to healthcare provider (HCP).
3. Encourage regular HCP visits to treat moles found in areas where there is friction or repeated irritation.

Important nursing interventions	Serious/life-threatening implications
Common signs & symptoms	Patient teaching

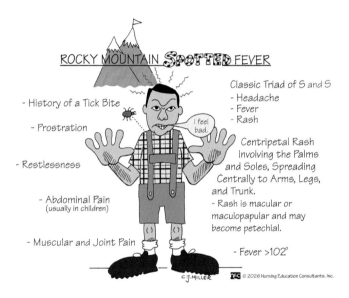

ROCKY MOUNTAIN SPOTTED FEVER

- History of a Tick Bite

- Prostration

- Restlessness

- Abdominal Pain
(usually in children)

- Muscular and Joint Pain

I feel bad.

Classic Triad of S and S
- Headache
- Fever
- Rash

Centripetal Rash Involving the Palms and Soles, Spreading Centrally to Arms, Legs, and Trunk.
- Rash is macular or maculopapular and may become petechial.

- Fever >102°

C.J. MILLER

Integumentary

What You Need to Know
Rocky Mountain Spotted Fever

DEFINITION

Rocky Mountain spotted fever (RMSF) is a tickborne disease caused by *Rickettsia rickettsia* and is the most lethal tick disease. The tick is found usually in the east of the Rocky Mountain region, and the vector is *Dermacentor variabilis* (dog tick).

COMPLICATIONS

- Meningoencephalitis, seizure, acute kidney injury
- Acute respiratory distress syndrome (ARDS), shock, arrhythmia

RECOGNIZE AND ANALYZE CUES

- Influenza-like symptoms in summer months
- Rapidly progressive disease without early treatment

MEDICAL MANAGEMENT: GENERATE SOLUTIONS

- Drugs: doxycycline
- Medication is started immediately without waiting for confirmation because of increased morbidity and mortality rate

NURSING MANAGEMENT: TAKE ACTION

1. Assess for recent tick bite, which is often painless; determine possible exposure to areas where ticks are found and travel history (where RMSF is endemic).
2. Teach protective measures:
   - Avoid dogs with ticks and tick-infected areas.
   - Use protective, light-colored clothing that covers arms and legs; tuck pants in socks to protect legs.
   - Apply tick-repellent chemicals such as DEET or permethrin to pants and sleeves.
   - Examine the entire body every 3 to 4 hours when in an infested area.

Important nursing interventions   Serious/life-threatening implications

Common signs & symptoms   Patient teaching

TIPS ON HEALING WOUNDS

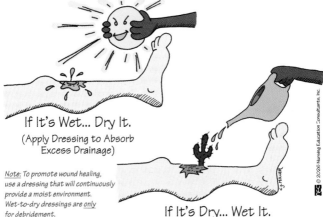

If It's Wet... Dry It.
(Apply Dressing to Absorb
Excess Drainage)

Note: To promote wound healing,
use a dressing that will continuously
provide a moist environment.
Wet-to-dry dressings are *only*
for debridement.

If It's Dry... Wet It.
(Apply a Moist Dressing)

What You Need to Know
Tips on Healing Wounds

DEFINITION

A wound involves a break or opening in the skin and occurs because of surgery, accidents, or injuries. Wounds can be minor such as a scrape or cut and can be deep involving bones, blood vessels, and nerves.

COMPLICATIONS OF HEALING

- Infection, hemorrhage, fistula formation
- Keloid formation, hypertrophic scars
- Adhesions, contractions, dehiscence, evisceration

STAGES OF WOUND HEALING

Wounds heal in stages. The smaller the wound, the faster the healing.
- Primary intention
  - Takes place when wound margins are approximated
  - Involves four phases that overlap—hemostasis (stop bleeding); inflammation (new framework for blood vessel growth); proliferation or granulation (wound pulls closed); and remodeling or maturation (formation of scar)
- Secondary intention
  - Involves a large wound area with irregular margins
  - Heals with larger scar due to larger amount of granulation tissue formed
- Tertiary intention
  - Delayed primary intention healing after 4 to 6 days
  - Occurs when contaminated wound is left open and sutured after the infection has healed
  - Involves a larger, deeper scar

NURSING MANAGEMENT: TAKE ACTION

1. Protect wounds from further trauma; prevent infection.
2. Keep wounds clean during the granulating and reepithelializing phase and slightly moist.
3. Prevent a wound from drying out because dryness will interfere with healing. Do not "air out" a wound because wounds need a moist environment to heal.
4. Apply an absorptive dressing to wounds that have excess drainage to draw the drainage away from the wound surface to allow healing to occur.

Important nursing interventions	Serious/life-threatening implications
Common signs & symptoms	Patient teaching

CATARACT

Characteristics

Cloudy, opaque lens

↓ Visual Acuity

Glare due to light
scatter on lens

Occurs gradually

↓ Night Vision

No pain

Treatment

Removal of lens with
lens implant

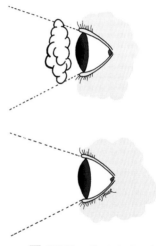

© 2026 Nursing Education Consultants, Inc.

What You Need to Know
Cataract

DEFINITION

A cataract is a complete or partial opacity of the lens that compromises the sharpness of images on the retina. It may occur at birth (congenital cataract) but is most common in adults past middle age (senile cataracts).

RISK FACTORS

- Diabetes mellitus, hypertension, advanced age
- Corticosteroids: long-term systemic or topical use, alcohol, tobacco use
- Trauma to the eye, exposure to radioactive materials, ultraviolet radiation

COMPLICATIONS

- Hemorrhage, infection, or ↑intraocular pressure (IOP)

RECOGNIZE AND ANALYZE CUES

- ↓Decreased visual acuity, blurred vision → double vision
- ↓Color perception, glaring, distortion, or "ghosting" of images

MEDICAL MANAGEMENT: GENERATE SOLUTIONS

- Nonsurgical: corrective lenses, increased lighting
- Drugs: mydriatics before surgery
- Surgery: phacoemulsification (most common) with lens implant, extracapsular extraction

NURSING MANAGEMENT: TAKE ACTION

1. Anticipate discharge after anesthetic agent wears off.
2. Teach about postoperative care and provide written instructions—how to instill eye drops, avoid rubbing or scratching the eye, recognizing symptoms of complications (severe eye pain, ↑redness of eye, drainage from eye, ↓vision in eye).

Important nursing interventions	Serious/life-threatening implications
Common signs & symptoms	Patient teaching

GLAUCOMA

* Increased Intraocular Pressure & Progressive Vision Loss *

Risk Factors - Familial
- Family History
- Over Age 40
- Diabetes, Hypertension

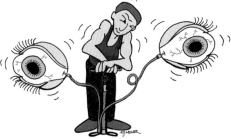

Primary Open-Angle Glaucoma (POAG)

- Gradual Loss of
  Peripheral Vision
  (Tunnel Vision)

- Generally Painless

- Blindness if Untreated

- ↓Visual Acuity

- ↑IOP>22 mm Hg

What You Need to Know
Glaucoma

DEFINITION

Glaucoma is a group of disorders characterized by an increase in intraocular pressure (IOP), optic nerve atrophy, and progressive loss of peripheral vision. It is an acute or chronic condition and a leading cause of blindness that can be prevented with early detection/treatment.

RISK FACTORS

- Family history, aging

COMPLICATIONS

- Loss of peripheral vision, blindness

RECOGNIZE AND ANALYZE CUES

- Two types of glaucoma
  - Primary angle-closure glaucoma (PACG, acute)—sudden, severe eye pain, nausea, vomiting with rapid ↑IOP; blindness occurs if not treated immediately
  - Primary open-angle glaucoma (POAG, chronic)—more common, slow onset, progressive loss of peripheral vision
  - Diagnostic: ↑IOP >22 mm Hg

MEDICAL MANAGEMENT: GENERATE SOLUTIONS

- Drugs: prostaglandin analogues (latanoprost, travoprost, bimatoprost); β-adrenergic blocker (timolol); α-adrenergic agonists (brimonidine); carbonic anhydrase inhibitors (acetazolamide); miotics (pilocarpine); hyperosmotic agent (mannitol); Rho kinase (Rock) inhibitors (netarsudil)
- Surgery: argon laser trabeculoplasty, trabeculectomy with or without filtering implant
- PACG: laser peripheral iridotomy, surgical iridectomy

NURSING MANAGEMENT: TAKE ACTION

1. Teach how to administer eye medications.
2. Teach the importance of having vision and IOP monitored frequently.
3. Anticipate early discharge from any operative procedure (usually done outpatient); provide written postoperative instructions.

CORNEAL TRANSPLANT SURGERY

You're Invited To The After Care Party Following CORNEAL TRANSPLANT SURGERY...

Watch For:

R. Redness
S. Swelling
V. Vision decrease
P. Pain

DANGER

DRAINAGE & REJECTION
- PURULENT DRAINAGE -
Signs of Infection

— Sensitivity to Light; Feeling of a Speck of Sand in the Eye —
Signs of Rejection

C.J. MILLER

What You Need to Know
Corneal Transplant Surgery

DEFINITION

Corneal transplant (keratoplasty) is the surgical removal of diseased corneal tissue and replacement with tissue from a human donor cornea.

INDICATIONS FOR SURGERY

- Corneal problems—keratoconus (degeneration of anterior corneal tissue resulting in an abnormal cone shape, which bulges forward)
- Eye injury, ulceration, keratitis, scarring

COMPLICATIONS

- Bleeding, wound leakage, infection, graft rejection

NURSING MANAGEMENT: TAKE ACTION

1. Explain the importance of wearing eye shields or glasses as prescribed.
2. Encourage patient to sleep on back rather than on the side.
3. Teach how to administer eye drops; avoid rubbing or pressing the eye.
4. Teach to monitor for symptoms of rejection of the cornea transplant—loss of vision, eye pain, red eyes, and sensitivity to light.
5. Stress the importance of frequent follow-up exams.

Important nursing interventions	Serious/life-threatening implications
Common signs & symptoms	Patient teaching

HEARING LOSS TYPES AND CAUSES

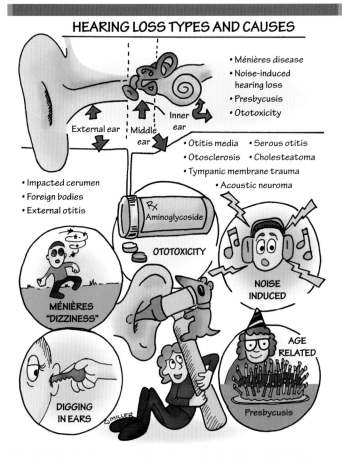

- Ménières disease
- Noise-induced hearing loss
- Presbycusis
- Ototoxicity

External ear | Middle ear | Inner ear

- Otitis media
- Serous otitis
- Otosclerosis
- Cholesteatoma
- Tympanic membrane trauma
- Acoustic neuroma

- Impacted cerumen
- Foreign bodies
- External otitis

Rx Aminoglycoside

OTOTOXICITY

NOISE INDUCED

MÉNIÈRES "DIZZINESS"

DIGGING IN EARS

AGE RELATED

Presbycusis

C. MILLER

What You Need to Know
Causes of Hearing Loss

DEFINITION

Hearing loss is a decrease in the ability to perceive and comprehend sound and can be partial, complete, unilateral, and/or bilateral. Typically, it is defined as a deficit of greater than 25 dB. Normal hearing is in the 0- to 15-dB range.

TYPES OF HEARING LOSS

- *Conductive* hearing loss occurs when outer or middle ear problems impair the transmission of sound waves to the inner ear.
  - Common causes: impacted cerumen (earwax); otitis media; tympanic membrane perforation; otosclerosis; allergies; benign tumors
- *Sensorineural* hearing loss is caused by damage to the inner ear or the vestibulocochlear nerve (CN VIII).
  - Common causes: congenital and hereditary factors; noise exposure; aging (presbycusis); Ménière disease; trauma; ototoxicity (aminoglycosides, NSAIDs)
- *Mixed* hearing loss occurs from a combination of conductive and sensorineural damage.
- *Central* hearing loss involves the inability to interpret sound, including speech, because of a problem in the brain or central nervous system.
- *Functional* hearing loss is often due to an emotional or psychological factor.

RECOGNIZE AND ANALYZE CUES

- Early signs of hearing loss—answering questions inappropriately and not responding when not looking at the speaker; often not aware of degree of hearing loss, especially if it is minimal hearing loss due to insidious onset and slow progression
- Bilateral tinnitus (ringing in the ears); often first symptom in older adult
- Straining to hear, cupping the hand around the ear, reading lips, being sensitive to slight increases in noise level
- Sudden deafness or rapid hearing loss in one ear is a medical emergency
- Diagnostics: audiometry, tuning fork test, CT scan, MRI

Important nursing interventions	Serious/life-threatening implications
Common signs & symptoms	Patient teaching

ANAPHYLACTIC REACTION

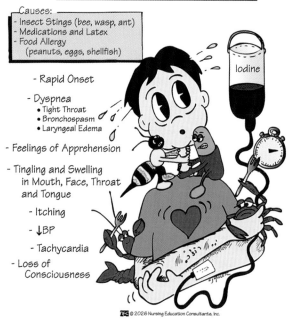

Causes:
- Insect Stings (bee, wasp, ant)
- Medications and Latex
- Food Allergy
  (peanuts, eggs, shellfish)

- Rapid Onset

- Dyspnea
  • Tight Throat
  • Bronchospasm
  • Laryngeal Edema

- Feelings of Apprehension

- Tingling and Swelling
  in Mouth, Face, Throat
  and Tongue

  - Itching

  - ↓BP

  - Tachycardia

- Loss of
  Consciousness

Iodine

© 2026 Nursing Education Consultants, Inc.

What You Need to Know
Anaphylactic Reaction

DEFINITION

Anaphylaxis is a type I, IgE-mediated sudden reaction that occurs in patients who are highly sensitized to a specific allergen—medications, blood products, insect stings. The antigen-antibody response precipitates the release of histamine, causing vasodilation and increased capillary permeability, which can be life threatening.

RISK FACTORS

- Antibiotics, injectable contrast media (dyes), vaccines
- Insect stings, allergies to foods, blood products

RECOGNIZE AND ANALYZE CUES

- The more rapid the onset of symptoms after exposure, the more severe the reaction
- Review figure

COMPLICATIONS

- Related to delay in treatment—dysrhythmias, shock, cardiopulmonary arrest

MEDICAL MANAGEMENT: GENERATE SOLUTIONS

- Drugs: parenteral epinephrine (IM, IV); nebulized albuterol for bronchospasm; IV corticosteroids; IV diphenhydramine for hives and itching

NURSING MANAGEMENT: TAKE ACTION

1. Manage a medical emergency by early recognition of signs and symptoms of an anaphylactic reaction.
2. Maintain a patent airway; high flow oxygen (8–10 L/min) via face mask; anticipate use of airway adjuncts (tracheostomy, endotracheal intubation).
3. Administer medications and treat shock.
   - For hypotension place recumbent and elevate legs; administer IV normal saline rapid bolus of 1 to 2 L.
   - Maintain blood pressure (BP) with fluids, volume expanders, vasopressors (e.g., dopamine).
4. Teach about the importance of avoiding known allergens whenever possible, wearing a medical alert bracelet, alerting healthcare personnel (HCP) about specific allergies.
5. Teach how to use an automatic epinephrine injector and to always have it with them.

Important nursing interventions	Serious/life-threatening implications
Common signs & symptoms	Patient teaching

SYSTEMIC LUPUS ERYTHEMATOSUS (SLE)

- Tachypnea
- Cough
- Pleural Inflammation/ Effusion

Photo-sensitivity

- Weight Loss
- Chronic Fatigue
- Fever—↑Risk of Infection
- Polyarthritis
- Emotional Lability
- Hematologic Disorders
- Coagulation Problems
- CNS Disorders— Seizures

Butterfly Rash Over Cheeks

C.J. MILLER

Dysrhythmias

Raynaud Phenomenon

Pericarditis

Vascular Inflammation

Glomerulonephritis —

Proteinuria –

Hematuria —

Immune

What You Need to Know

Systemic Lupus Erythematosus (SLE)

DEFINITION

SLE is a multisystem inflammatory autoimmune disorder that affects multiple organs and is characterized by a diffuse production of autoantibodies that form immune complexes that attack and cause damage to body organs and tissue.

RISK FACTORS

- More common in females 20 to 40 years of age; familial tendencies
- More prevalent in Black populations, Asian, Hispanic, and Native Americans than in White Americans
- May be triggered by environmental stimulus, infections, and medications; sun exposure is most common

COMPLICATIONS

- Kidney failure, cardiovascular and thromboembolic events, infections, death

RECOGNIZE AND ANALYZE CUES

- Severity of symptoms varies greatly throughout the course of the disease; periods of exacerbation (flares) and remission occur
- Diagnostics: ↑antinuclear antibody titer (ANA), ↑estimated sedimentation rate (ESR), ↑C-reactive protein (CRP); testing for anti-DNA antibodies, anti-Smith (Sm) antibodies, antiphospholipid antibodies

MEDICAL MANAGEMENT: GENERATE SOLUTIONS

- Drugs: hydroxychloroquine; corticosteroids for flares; NSAIDs; methotrexate; immunosuppressives (cyclophosphamide, azathioprine); topical immunomodulators (tacrolimus, pimecrolimus) to treat skin problems
- Focus is on preventing flares and end-organ damage

NURSING MANAGEMENT: TAKE ACTION

1. Anticipate problems of persistent pain, chronic inflammation, fatigue, potential loss of tissue integrity, decreased self-esteem owing to body image changes.
2. Teach about signs and symptoms to report to HCP (e.g., fever, edema, ↓urine output, chest pain, dyspnea).
3. Teach about the importance of adherence to medication therapy and lifestyle changes (avoiding sunlight) to prevent exacerbations.

HUMAN IMMUNODEFICIENCY VIRUS (HIV) INFECTION

Transmission:

- Unprotected Sexual Intercourse
- Contact with Blood and Blood Products
- Perinatal—during pregnancy, delivery, or breastfeeding

Types of HIV Tests

- Antibody tests—detects only antibodies
- Antigen/antibody tests—detects both
- Nucleic acid tests (NAT)—detects the HIV virus

Seroconversion – development of HIV—**specific antibodies**

- Window Period—typically 3 weeks between infection and detection of antibodies (HIV positive)

Acquired Immunodeficiency Disease Syndrome – (AIDS) presence of at least

one or more:

- CD4 Tcell count ↓200 cells/uL **(compromised immune system)**
- Opportunistic infections –
  Fungal – **Candidiasis, Pneunocystis jiroveci pneumonia (PCP)**
  Viral – **Cytomegalovirus (CMV)**
  Bacterial – **Mycobacterium tuberculosis, pneumonia**
  Protozoal – **Toxoplasmosis of brain, intestine**
- Cancer
  Invasive Cervical Cancer
  Kaposi sarcoma
  Lymphoma
  Burkitt lymphoma
- Wasting Syndrome

| **Acute HIV Infection** |
- Occurs about 2–4 weeks after infected
- Symptoms (flu-like)—fever, chills, swollen lymph nodes, sore throat, mouth ulcers, night sweats, fatigue, nausea, muscle aches, joint pain, diffuse rash
- High viral load

| **Chronic Infection** |
- May have asymptomatic infection, can still transmit infection
- May be symptomatic as the CD4 cell count declines closer to 200 cells/μL and the viral load increases
- Infections occur

| **AIDS** |
- Meets Criteria for AIDS Diagnosis

Treatment:

- Antiretroviral therapy (ART) begins with confirmation of HIV (lifelong therapy)

Goals:

- Decrease viral load
- Maintain or ↑CD4+ T-Cell count
- Delay onset of HIV-related symptoms
- Prevent or delay opportunistic infections

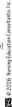

© 2026 Nursing Education Consultants, Inc.

What You Need to Know

Human Immunodeficiency Virus (HIV) Infection

DEFINITION

HIV is a virus that attacks the body's immune system. If HIV is not treated, it can lead to AIDS (acquired immunodeficiency syndrome). There is currently no effective cure. Once people get HIV, they have it for life.

RECOGNIZE AND ANALYZE CUES

- Review figure
- Diagnostics: the *window period* is the time between a potential HIV exposure and an accurate test result; each HIV test has their own window period
  - Positive test result means the person has HIV—it does not predict the course of the disease
  - Negative test result means that HIV antibodies were not detected, but this can occur during the window period of seroconversion

MEDICAL MANAGEMENT: GENERATE SOLUTIONS

- Drugs: antiretroviral (ART) therapy; used with a combination of two to three ART drugs (lifelong therapy)
  - PrEP (pre-exposure prophylaxis) is medication for people at risk for HIV but who do not have HIV. PrEP is highly effective for preventing HIV from sex or injection drug use.
  - PEP (postexposure prophylaxis) must be started within 72 hours after possible exposure (needlestick, sexual exposure, sexual assault); need to take medication daily for 28 days
  - Preventive vaccines (hepatitis A, hepatitis B, influenza, pneumococcal)

NURSING MANAGEMENT: TAKE ACTION

1. Provide information on how HIV is transmitted and preventive measures.
   - HIV *cannot* be transmitted by hugging, kissing, holding hands, or other non-sexual contact; from inanimate objects (money, doorknobs, bathtubs, toilet seats, etc.); from dishes, silverware, or food handled by an infected person; or by animals or insects.
   - Explain risk-reducing sexual activities, how to reduce the risk related to drug abuse, perinatal transmission, occupational exposure (healthcare workers).
   - Teach the importance of detecting HIV infection *early*.
2. Promote health during the acute stage of HIV infection.
3. Monitor for opportunistic problems caused by HIV infection.

Important nursing interventions	Serious/life-threatening implications
Common signs & symptoms	Patient teaching

TYPES OF DISASTERS

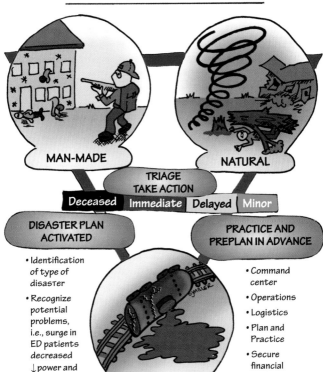

MAN-MADE

NATURAL

TRIAGE TAKE ACTION

Deceased | Immediate | Delayed | Minor

DISASTER PLAN ACTIVATED

PRACTICE AND PREPLAN IN ADVANCE

- Identification of type of disaster
- Recognize potential problems, i.e., surge in ED patients decreased ↓power and resources

- Command center
- Operations
- Logistics
- Plan and Practice
- Secure financial backing

TECHNOLOGICAL

What You Need to Know
Types of Disasters

DEFINITION

There are three categories of disaster levels for nurses that identify the extent of nursing intervention needed, the number of resources needed, and the expected duration of response: *natural, man-made*, and *technological*.

RISK FACTORS

- Level of threat to life
- Geographic area involved
- Weather
- Hospital resources
- Frequency/predictability of event

CHARACTERISTICS OF DISASTERS

- Frequency—how often does it occur?
  - *Example*: tornadoes most often occur in the spring and fall
- Predictability—having the ability to determine when and where the disaster might occur
  - *Example*: flooding can be predicted in the spring following a snowmelt
- Preventability/mitigation—what actions can be taken before the disaster happens to lessen the loss of life and property damage?
  - *Example:* some disasters (e.g., hurricanes, tornadoes, earthquakes) are not preventable; flooding can be controlled through dams or levees
- Imminence—what is the speed of onset of the disaster related to forewarning and the anticipated duration of the event?
  - *Example*: weather forecasters can provide projections of when a tornado or hurricane may occur; wildfires, explosions, or terrorist attacks cannot be predicted
- Scope and number of casualties—involves the geographic area and the number of individuals affected
  - *Example*: earthquakes and tsunamis may involve many people or a smaller number if adequate preventive measures are in place
- Intensity—what is the level of destruction and devastation from the disaster?
  - *Example*: availability of scales to measure events such as the Enhanced Fujita Scale (EF Scale) for tornadoes or the Saffir-Simpson Hurricane Scale (category 1 to category 5 [most catastrophic]) for hurricanes

DISASTER MANAGEMENT

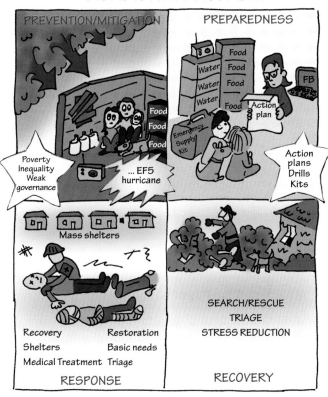

What You Need to Know
Disaster Management

DEFINITION

Disaster management is a four-stage circular cycle involving *Prevention (Mitigation)*, *Preparedness*, *Response*, and *Recovery*. Nurses must possess a unique skillset for each stage, which may include assessment, priority setting, collaboration, and health education.

RISK FACTORS

- Environmental degradation (climate change)
- Globalized economic development
- Poverty and inequality
- Weak governance
- Epidemics/pandemics

COMPLICATIONS

- Mass casualties
- Vulnerable populations
- Psychological stress
  - Individual/community
  - Disaster workers/first responders

RECOGNIZE AND ANALYZE CUES

- Epidemiology and surveillance of disaster-related syndromes and maladies
- Surge in hospital census counts
- Emergency activation (government disaster declaration, emergency operations center)
- Social media and mobile technology communications

MEDICAL MANAGEMENT: GENERATE SOLUTIONS

- Implement Incident Command System (ICS) for events
- Strategic National Stockpile
- Disaster Medical Assistance Teams (DMAT)
- Individual/Community Preparedness

NURSING MANAGEMENT: TAKE ACTION

1. Strengthen/sustain health and emergency response systems.
2. Build individual and community preparedness and resilience.
3. Triage.
4. Perform routine drills and exercising.
5. Reduce stress in individuals during disasters.
6. Sheltering operations for people displaced by disasters.

Important nursing interventions	Serious/life-threatening implications
Common signs & symptoms	Patient teaching

TRIAGE

Keep Calm and Triage On. . . .
Rehearsed Emergency Plans and
Sorting Patients According
to Medical Need

DECEASED

NOT VIABLE

IMMEDIATE

FIRST PRIORITY

INJURIES NEEDING ADVANCED CARE

Remember your A - B - C s

DELAYED

WALKING WOUNDED, THOSE NEEDING
SUTURES, TREATMENTS, WOUND CARE

MINOR

SCRAPES   SPRAINS   EMOTIONAL   TRAUMA

===== **What You Need to Know** =====
Triage

DEFINITION
Triage is a system of categorizing patients according to medical need when resources are unavailable for all persons to be treated.

RISK FACTORS
- Mass casualty incident
  - Natural disaster—tornado, hurricane, blizzard, flash flooding
  - Man-made disaster—active shooter, plane crash, civilian bombing, chemical release
  - Technological disaster—chemical spill, transportation accidents, fires/explosions
- Epidemic/pandemic of emerging or reemerging infectious disease (COVID-19)

COMPLICATIONS
- Availability of hospital resources
- Bed availability

RECOGNIZE AND ANALYZE CUES
- Surge in patients presenting to emergency department with similar symptoms
- Man-made disaster (e.g., sporting event bombing, plane crash)
- Hospital Incident Command System (HICS) or Hospital Emergency Incident Command System (HEICS) activation

NURSING MANAGEMENT: TAKE ACTION
1. Remember the ABCs.
2. Implement START triage tags/categorization:
   - **DECEASED** (Black card)—Injury beyond scope of medical assistance. Tag only if they are not breathing and attempts to resuscitate have been unsuccessful.
   - **IMMEDIATE** (Red card)—Injury can be assisted or health aided by advanced medical care <1 hour.
   - **DELAYED** (Yellow card)—Injury assisted after "Immediate" persons. Medically stable but require medical assistance.
   - **MINOR** (Green card)—Injury assisted after "Immediate" and "Delayed." Injury can wait several hours and injured can walk without assistance.
3. Knowledge of appropriate pharmacological therapies for biological, chemical, and radiologic agents.
4. Practice triage training by performing tabletop drills and functional exercises using triage tags with hospital staff.

Important nursing interventions	Serious/life-threatening implications
Common signs & symptoms	Patient teaching

EMERGENCY RESPONSE PLAN

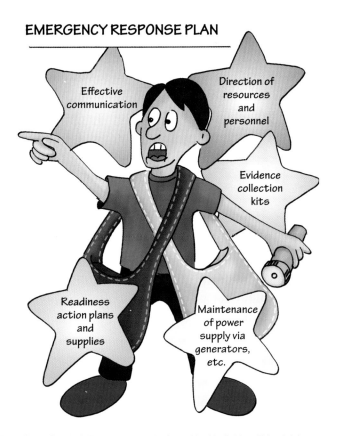

What You Need to Know
Emergency Response Plan

DEFINITION

A set of written procedures for dealing with emergencies that minimizes the impact of event and facilitates recovery. These plans facilitate and organize employer and employee actions during workplace emergencies and disasters.

LOCAL GOVERNMENTAL RESPONSIBILITIES

- *First responders* (e.g., police, fire, public health, public works, emergency services) are responsible for incident management
- Manage incidents by carrying out evacuation, search and rescue, maintaining public health and public works
- Communication from first responders and others to the *Office of Emergency Management* determines what other resources are needed

STATE GOVERNMENTAL RESPONSIBILITIES

- Become involved when community sources are overwhelmed and the state's *Department or Office of Emergency Management* is called for assistance
- *National Response Framework* is the core operational plan for domestic incident management for an all-hazards response

FEDERAL GOVERNMENTAL RESPONSIBILITIES

- *US Department of Homeland Security* focuses on protecting the American people and their homeland
- *Federal Emergency Management Agency (FEMA)* supports community and first responders to prepare, protect, respond, recover, and mitigate all hazards
- *Centers for Disease Control and Prevention* (CDC) ensures that there is clean drinking water, food, shelter, and medical care available for disaster victims

---

Important nursing interventions

Serious/life-threatening implications

Common signs & symptoms

Patient teaching

Note: Page numbers followed by *f* indicate figures.

–A–

ABCDEs. *See* Airway, breathing, circulation, disability, exposure
Acetylcholine, 172
Acquired immunodeficiency syndrome (AIDS), 239*f*, 240
Acromegaly
  clinical manifestations, 1*f*
  complications, 1*f*, 2
  definition, 1*f*, 2
  diagnosis, 1*f*
  medical management, 2
  nursing management, 2–3
  recognize and analyze cues, 2
Acute blood transfusion reactions
  definition, 40
  medical management, 40
  nursing management, 40–41
  recognize and analyze cues, 40
  types, 39*f*
Acute decompensated heart failure (ADHF), 98, 100, 102
Acute hemolytic, blood transfusion reaction, 44
Acute kidney injury (AKI)
  phases
    complications, 210
    definition, 210
    medical management, 210

Acute kidney injury (AKI) *(Continued)*
    nursing management, 210–212
    recognize and analyze cues, 210
    signs and symptoms, 209*f*
  stages
    causes, 208
    definition, 208
    intrarenal, 208
    postrenal, 208
    prerenal, 208
    recognize and analyze cues, 208–210
    RIFLE, 207*f*, 208
Acute lymphocytic leukemia, 50
Acute myeloid leukemia, 50
Acute pancreatitis, 139*f*, 140
Acute peripheral neuropathy, 168
Acute respiratory distress syndrome (ARDS)
  causes, 71*f*
  complications, 72
  definition, 72
  medical management, 72
  nursing management, 72–73
  recognize and analyze cues, 72
  risk factors, 72
  signs and symptoms, 71*f*
Acute thyrotoxicosis, 6

Acute tubular necrosis (ATN), 208

AD. *See* Autonomic dysreflexia

Addison disease
  complications, 30
  definition, 30
  medical management, 30
  nursing management, 30–31
  recognize and analyze cues, 30
  risk factors, 30
  symptoms, 29f

ADH. *See* Antidiuretic hormone

ADHF. *See* Acute decompensated
     heart failure

Adrenal cortex, 34
  glucocorticoids, 34
  mineralocorticoids, 34
  sex hormones, 34

Adrenal crisis, 29f, 30

Adrenalectomy, 32

Adrenal gland hormones
  cortex, 34
  definition, 34
  medulla, 34

Adrenal medulla, 34
  dopamine, 34
  epinephrine, 34
  norepinephrine, 34

Adrenocortical insufficiency, 29f

Adrenocorticotropic hormone (ACTH)
  simulation test, 30

Aging, 58

AIDS. *See* Acquired immunodeficiency
    syndrome

Airway, breathing, circulation, disability,
    exposure (ABCDEs), 172

AKI. *See* Acute kidney injury

Aldosterone, 34

Allergic (anaphylactic)
  acute transfusion reactions, 39f, 40
  blood transfusion reaction, 44

Alpha$_1$-antitrypsin deficiency, 58

ALS. *See* Amyotrophic lateral sclerosis

Alternative ventilation strategies, 72

American College of Cardiology, 98

American Heart Association, 98, 150

Aminocaproic acid, 46

Amyotrophic lateral sclerosis (ALS)
  definition, 164
  medical management, 164
  nursing management, 163f, 164–166
  recognize and analyze cues, 164
  risk factors, 164

Anaphylactic, blood transfusion
    reaction, 44

Anaphylactic reaction. *See* Anaphylaxis

Anaphylactic shock, 92

Anaphylaxis
  causes, 235f
  complications, 236
  definition, 236
  medical management, 236
  nursing management, 236–237
  recognize and analyze cues, 236
  risk factors, 236
  symptoms, 235f

Androstenedione, 34

Anemia
  aplastic, 36
  complications, 36
  definition, 36
  folic acid deficiency, 36
  iron deficiency, 36
  medical management, 36
  nursing management, 36–37
  recognize and analyze cues, 36
  types, 35f
  vitamin B$_{12}$ deficiency, 36
Anticoagulant therapy, 64
Antidiabetic drugs, 18
Antidiuretic hormone (ADH), 4
Antigen-antibody response, 236
Antihypertensive agents, 80
Antiplatelet therapy, 96
Antiresorptive medications, 194
Antiretroviral (ART) therapy, 240
Aortic dissection
  complications, 90
  definition, 90
  medical management, 90
  nursing management, 90–92
  recognize and analyze cues, 90
  risk factors, 90
  symptoms, 89f
Aphasia, 152
Aplastic anemia, 36
Apneic episodes, 74
Appendicitis
  complications, 108
  definition, 108

Appendicitis (Continued)
  diagnosis, 107f
  medical management, 108
  nursing management, 108–110
  recognize and analyze cues, 108
  risk factors, 108
  symptoms, 107f
  treatment, 107f
Apraxia of speech, 152
ARDS. See Acute respiratory distress
      syndrome
Arterial versus venous ulcers, 85f
Asthma
  attack, 53f
  complications, 54
  definition, 54
  emergency, 53f
  medical management, 54
  nursing management, 54–55
  recognize and analyze cues, 54
  risk factors/triggers, 53f, 54
Asthma-COPD overlap syndrome, 58
Atherosclerosis, progression of
  definition, 78
  medical management, 78
  modifiable risk factors, 78
  nonmodifiable risk factors, 78
  nursing management, 78–80
  recognize and analyze cues, 78
  symptoms, 77f
ATN. See Acute tubular necrosis
Autoantibodies, 238
Autoimmune disorders, 30, 168

Autonomic dysreflexia (AD)
    complications, 160
    definition, 160
    nursing management, 160–162
    recognize and analyze cues, 160
    risk factors, 160
    symptoms, 159f
Autonomic nervous system, 168

–B–

Bacterial contamination (septic), blood
        transfusion reaction, 44
Barnett Continent Intestinal Reservoir,
        116
Basilar skull fracture, 142
Bell palsy
    complications, 174
    definition, 174
    etiology, 173f
    medical management, 174
    nursing management, 174–176
    recognize and analyze cues,
        174
    risk factors, 174
    treatment, 173f
Benign prostatic hyperplasia (BPH),
        202. See also Transurethral
        resection of the prostate
Bilateral tinnitus, 234
Bilevel positive airway pressure
        (BiPAP), 66
Bisphosphonates, 194

Blood administration. See Blood
        transfusion
Blood glucose
    definition, 14
    medications, 14
    nursing management, 14–15
    recognize and analyze cues, 14
    symptoms, 13f
Blood osmolarity, 22
Blood sugar. See Blood glucose
Blood transfusion
    acute reactions. See Acute blood
        transfusion reactions
    complications, 38
    definition, 38
    delayed reactions. See Delayed
        blood transfusion reactions
    elements, 37f
    medical management, 38
    nursing management, 38–39, 43f,
        44–45
        after responsibilities, 38–39
        before responsibilities, 38
        during responsibilities, 38
Bone mineral density (BMD), 192
Borrelia burgdorferi, 220
Bowel obstruction
    complications, 112
    definition, 112
    medical management, 112
    nursing management, 112–114
    recognize and analyze cues, 112
    risk factors, 112

Bowel obstruction *(Continued)*
  symptoms, 111*f*
  types of, 113*f*, 114
    complications, 114
    definition, 114
    mechanical, 114
    nonmechanical, 114
    recognize and analyze cues,
      114–116
    risk factors, 114
BPH. *See* Benign prostatic hyperplasia
Brain attack. *See* Stroke
Brain mass, 144
Breast cancer, 200
Bronchial mucosa, 62
Buck's traction, 182
Burn depth. *See* Depth of burns

–C–

Calcium oxalate, 206
Calcium phosphate, 206
Calcium supplements, 194
Cardiac resynchronization therapy
    (CRT), 100
Cardiac tamponade, 92
Cardiogenic shock, 92
Care of patient in traction
  definition, 183*f*, 184
  nursing implications, 184–186
  types of, 184
Cast application/splinting, fracture,
    180

Cataract
  characteristics, 227*f*
  complications, 228
  definition, 228
  medical management, 228
  nursing management, 228–229
  recognize and analyze cues, 228
  risk factors, 228
  treatment, 227*f*
Catheter-associated urinary tract
    infections, 204–206
Centers for Disease Control and
    Prevention, 248
Central (neurogenic) DI, 3*f*, 4
Central hearing loss, 234
Central herniation, 144
Cerebral edema, 20, 22, 144
Cerebral herniation, 144
Cerebral vascular accident (CVA)
  functioning *versus* affected.
      See Functioning *versus* affected
      CVA
  left. *See* Left CVA
  right. *See* Right CVA
Cerebrospinal fluid (CSF), mustache
    dressing (drip pad), 2
Chest physiotherapy, 56
Chlorhexidine gluconate (CHG),
    190
Cholecystitis
  complications, 136
  definition, 136
  medical management, 136

Cholecystitis *(Continued)*
  nursing management, 136–138
  recognize and analyze cues, 136
  risk factors, 136
  symptoms, 135*f*
Cholinergic crisis, 170
  complications, 172
  definition, 172
  medical management, 172
  nursing management, 172–174
  recognize and analyze cues, 172
  risk factors, 172
  symptoms, 171*f*
Chronic arterial obstruction, 86
Chronic bronchitis, 58
  complications, 62
  definition, 62
  medical management, 62
  nursing management, 62–63
  recognize and analyze cues, 62
  risk factors, 62
  symptoms, 61*f*
Chronic HF, 98, 100, 102
Chronic illness, 218
Chronic kidney disease (CKD)
  definition, 212
  medical management, 212
  nursing management, 212–214
  recognize and analyze cues, 212
  risk factors, 212
  signs and symptoms, 211*f*
Chronic lymphocytic leukemia, 50
Chronic myelogenous leukemia, 50

Chronic obstructive pulmonary disease
    (COPD)
  complications, 58
  definition, 58
  medical management, 58
  nursing management, 58–59
  recognize and analyze cues, 58
  risk factors, 58
  symptoms, 57*f*
Chronic pancreatitis, 139*f*, 140
Chronic stable angina
  characteristics, 93*f*
  complications, 94
  definition, 94
  medical management, 94
  nursing management, 94–95
  recognize and analyze cues, 94
  risk factors, 94
  triggers, 93*f*
Chronic venous insufficiency
    (CVI), 86
Cingulate herniation, 144
Cirrhosis
  clinical manifestations, 127*f*
  complications, 128
  definition, 128
  medical management, 128
  nursing management, 128–130
  recognize and analyze cues, 128
  risk factors, 128
Closed reduction, fracture, 180
Clostridium tetani, 178
Cognitive impairments, 152

Colostomy, 116

Compartment syndrome, 180

Complex partial seizures, 146

Conductive hearing loss, 234

Congenital cataract, 228

Congestive heart failure. *See* Left-sided heart failure

Conservative therapy, 128

Constipation, bowel elimination, 106

Continent urinary diversions, 216
  orthotopic neobladder, 216
  reservoir, 216

Continent urinary reservoir, 216

COPD. *See* Chronic obstructive pulmonary disease

Corneal transplant surgery
  complications, 232
  definition, 232
  indications for, 232
  nursing management, 232–233
  RSVP, 231*f*

Cor pulmonale, 102

Corticosteroids, 30, 34, 228
  therapy, 32

Cortisol, 34

COVID-19
  complications, 76
  definition, 76
  medical management, 76
  nursing management, 76
  recognize and analyze cues, 76

COVID-19 *(Continued)*
  risk factors, 76
  signs and symptoms, 75*f*

Crohn's disease
  complications, 121*f*, 122
  definition, 122
  medical management, 122
  nursing management, 122–124
  recognize and analyze cues, 122
  risk factors, 122
  symptoms, 121*f*

CRT. *See* Cardiac resynchronization therapy

CSF. *See* Cerebrospinal fluid

Cushing syndrome
  complications, 32
  definition, 32
  medical management, 32
  nursing management, 32–33
  recognize and analyze cues, 32
  risk factors, 32
  symptoms, 31*f*

Cushing triad
  complications, 144
  definition, 144
  recognize and analyze cues, 144–146
  risk factors, 144
  symptoms, 143*f*

CVA. *See* Cerebral vascular accident

CVI. *See* Chronic venous insufficiency

Cystine, 206

Cystitis, 203*f*, 204

–D–

DASH. *See* Dietary Approaches to Stop Hypertension
Deceased triage, 246
Deep brain stimulation, 162
Deep vein thrombosis (DVT), 88
Dehydroepiandrosterone, 34
Delayed blood transfusion reactions
  definition, 42
  medical management, 42
  nursing management, 42–43
  recognize and analyze cues, 42
  types, 41*f*
Delayed hemolytic reaction, 41*f*, 42
Delayed triage, 246
Demyelination, 166
Depth of burns
  classification, 217*f*, 218
  definition, 218
  extent of, 218
  factors, 218
  full-thickness, 218
  location of, 218
  partial-thickness, 218
  risk factors, 218–219
Dermacentor variabilis, 224
Desmopressin, 46
DEXA. *See* Dual-energy x-ray absorptiometry
Dexamethasone suppression test, 32
Diabetes insipidus (DI)
  central (neurogenic), 3*f*, 4
  complications, 4

Diabetes insipidus (DI) *(Continued)*
  definition, 4
  medical management, 4
  nursing management, 4–5
  recognize and analyze cues, 4
  risk factors, 4
  treatment, 3*f*
Diabetes management
  definition, 18
  diet, 17*f*, 18–19
  exercise, 17*f*, 18
  medication, 17*f*, 18
  nursing management, 18–19
Diabetes mellitus (DM)
  diagnosis
    definition, 16
    factors, 16
    methods, 15*f*
    nursing management, 16–17
  management
    definition, 18
    diet, 17*f*, 18–19
    exercise, 17*f*, 18
    medication, 17*f*, 18
    nursing management, 18–19
  type 1. *See* Type 1 diabetes mellitus
  type 2. *See* Type 2 diabetes mellitus
Diabetic fitness, exercise guide for
  definition, 26
  nursing management, 26–27
Diabetic ketoacidosis (DKA), 10, 12
  complications, 20
  definition, 20

Diabetic ketoacidosis (DKA)
(Continued)
  medical management, 20
  nursing management, 20–21
  prevention, 20–21
  recognize and analyze cues, 20
  risk factors, 20
  symptoms, 19*f*
Diarrhea, bowel elimination, 106
Diastolic HF, 100
Diet
  diabetes management, 17*f*, 18–19
  interventions, 18
  sources, 18
Dietary Approaches to Stop
    Hypertension (DASH), 82
Disaster management
  complications, 244
  definition, 244
  medical management, 244
  nursing management, 244–245
  phases, 243*f*
  recognize and analyze cues, 244
  risk factors, 244
Disasters
  characteristics, 242–243
    frequency, 242
    imminence, 242
    intensity, 242–243
    predictability, 242
    preventability/mitigation, 242
    scope and number of casualties, 242
  definition, 242

Disasters *(Continued)*
  management. *See* Disaster
    management
  risk factors, 242
  types of, 241*f*
Dissecting aneurysm. *See* Aortic
    dissection
Distributive shock, 92
Diuretic phase, 210
Diuretics, 80
DKA. *See* Diabetic ketoacidosis
DM. *See* Diabetes mellitus
Dopamine, 34
Dual-energy x-ray absorptiometry
    (DEXA), 192
Dumping syndrome
  complications, 124
  definition, 124
  medical management, 124
  nursing management, 124–126
  recognize and analyze cues, 124
  risk factors, 124
  symptoms, 123*f*
Duodenal ulcers, 119*f*, 120
DVT. *See* Deep vein thrombosis
Dysarthria, 152
Dysphagia, 152

–E–

Embolic stroke, 150
Emergency response plan
  definition, 247*f*, 248

Emergency response plan *(Continued)*
federal governmental responsibilities, 248
local governmental responsibilities, 248
state governmental responsibilities, 248
Emphysema, 58
complications, 60
definition, 60
medical management, 60
nursing management, 60–61
recognize and analyze cues, 60
risk factors, 60
symptoms, 59f
Endothelial damage, 88
Endotracheal intubation, 72
Enhanced Fujita Scale (EF Scale), 242
Enteritis. See Crohn's disease
Epilepsy. See Seizures
Epinephrine, 34
Escherichia coli, 204
Esophageal varices, 128
Esophagus, 118
Exercise, diabetes management, 17f, 18
External fixation, fracture, 180

–F–

Facial drooping, arm weakness, speech difficulties, and time (FAST), 149f, 150

FAST recognition of stroke
definition, 149f, 150
recognize and analyze cues, 150–152
types of, 150
Febrile (nonhemolytic)
acute transfusion reactions, 39f, 40
blood transfusion reaction, 44
Fecal-oral transmission, 134
Federal Emergency Management Agency, 248
Federal governmental responsibilities, 248
FibroTest, 132
"15–15 Rule", 24
First responders, 248
Flatulence, bowel elimination, 106
Focal onset seizures, 146
Folic acid deficiency anemia, 36
Fracture
classification, 179f
complications, 180
definition, 180
extremity, 180
hip. See Hip fracture
medical management, 180
nursing management, 180–182
recognize and analyze cues, 180
risk factors, 180
Functional hearing loss, 234
Functioning *versus* affected CVA
definition, 155f, 156
nursing management, 156–158

–G–

Gastric ulcers, 119*f*, 120
Gastroesophageal reflux disease (GERD)
   complications, 118
   definition, 118
   medical management, 118
   nursing management, 118–120
   recognize and analyze cues, 118
   risk factors, 117*f*, 118
   treatment, 117*f*
Gastrointestinal (GI) tract, 106
Generalized onset seizures, 146
Genetic inheritance pattern, 46
Genitourinary, menopause, 198
GERD. *See* Gastroesophageal reflux disease
Gestational diabetes, 14
GH. *See* Growth hormone
Gigantism, 2
Glaucoma
   complications, 230
   definition, 230
   medical management, 230
   nursing management, 230–231
   recognize and analyze cues, 230
   risk factors, 229*f*, 230
Glucocorticoids, 30, 32, 34
Glucose, 14. *See also* Blood glucose
Grading scale system, 130
Grand mal seizures. *See* Tonic-clonic seizures

Graves disease, 6
Growth hormone (GH), 2
Guillain-Barré syndrome
   causes, 167*f*
   complications, 168
   definition, 168
   medical management, 168
   nursing management, 168–170
   recognize and analyze cues, 168
   risk factors, 167*f*, 168

–H–

Halo sign, 2
Hardening of the arteries, 78
HAV. *See* Hepatitis A virus
HBV. *See* Hepatitis B virus
HCV. *See* Hepatitis C virus
HDV. *See* Hepatitis D virus
HE. *See* Hepatic encephalopathy
Headache, migraine symptoms. *See* Migraine headache symptoms
Healing skin lesions. *See* Healing wounds
Healing wounds
   complications, 226
   definition, 225*f*, 226
   nursing management, 226
   stages of, 226
      primary intention, 226
      secondary intention, 226
      tertiary intention, 226

Hearing loss
  causes, 233f
  definition, 234
  recognize and analyze cues, 234
  types of, 233f, 234
    central, 234
    conductive, 234
    functional, 234
    mixed, 234
    sensorineural, 234
Heart failure (HF)
  classification and staging, 98
  definition, 98
  FACES of, 97f
  left-sided. See Left-sided heart failure
  recognize and analyze cues, 98–99
  right-sided. See Right-sided heart failure
  treatment
    BANDAID, 104
    DAD BOND CLASH, 104
    definition, 104
    unload fast, 103f
Hemiparesis, 152, 154
Hemiplegia, 152, 154
Hemodynamic pressure monitoring, 72
Hemodynamic stability, 122
Hemoglobin (Hgb), 16, 36
Hemolytic, acute transfusion reactions, 39f, 40
Hemophilia
  complications, 46

Hemophilia (Continued)
  definition, 46
  medical management, 46
  nursing management, 46–47
  recognize and analyze cues, 46
  risk factors, 46
  symptoms, 45f
Hemophilia A, 46
Hemophilia B, 46
Hemorrhagic stroke, 150
Hemorrhoids, bowel elimination, 106
Hemothorax, 70
Hepatic cirrhosis. See Cirrhosis
Hepatic encephalopathy (HE)
  complications, 130
  definition, 130
  medical management, 130
  nursing management, 130–132
  recognize and analyze cues, 130
  risk factors, 130
  symptoms, 129f
Hepatitis
  complications, 132
  definition, 132
  HAV. See Hepatitis A virus
  HBV. See Hepatitis B virus
  HCV. See Hepatitis C virus
  HDV. See Hepatitis D virus
  HEV. See Hepatitis E virus
  medical management, 132
  mode of transmission, 132
  nursing management, 132–134
  recognize and analyze cues, 132

Hepatitis *(Continued)*
  types, 131*f*
Hepatitis A virus (HAV), 132
  definition, 133*f*, 134
  nursing management, 134–136
  recognize and analyze cues, 134
  risk factors, 134
Hepatitis B virus (HBV), 132
  nursing management, 134–136
  recognize and analyze cues, 134
  risk factors, 134
Hepatitis C virus (HCV), 132
Hepatitis D virus (HDV), 132
Hepatitis E virus (HEV), 132, 133*f*, 134
Hernia, 142
  complications, 126
  definition, 126
  medical management, 126
  nursing management, 126
  recognize and analyze cues, 126
  risk factors, 126
HEV. *See* Hepatitis E virus
HF. *See* Heart failure
HHS. *See* Hyperglycemic-
    hyperosmolar state
High blood pressure (BP). *See*
    Hypertension
High-density lipoprotein, 28
Hip fracture
  complications, 182
  definition, 181*f*, 182
  medical management, 182
  nursing management, 182–184

Hip fracture *(Continued)*
  recognize and analyze cues, 182
  risk factors, 182
Homonymous hemianopia, 152, 154
Human immunodeficiency virus (HIV)
    infection
  goals, 239*f*
  treatment, 239*f*
Hydration, 122
Hypercoagulability, 88
Hypercortisolism. *See* Cushing
    syndrome
Hyperglycemia, 14, 28
Hyperglycemic-hyperosmolar state
    (HHS), 10, 12
  complications, 22
  definition, 22
  medical management, 22
  nursing management, 22–23
  recognize and analyze cues, 22
  risk factors, 22
  symptoms, 21*f*
Hypertension, 28
  complications, 80
  definition, 80
  medical management, 80–82
  nursing care
    definition, 82
    diuretic, 81*f*
    management, 82–84
  recognize and analyze cues, 80
  risk factors, 80
  types, 79*f*

Hypertensive crisis
  causes, 83f
  complications, 83f, 84
  definition, 84
  medical management, 84
  nursing management, 84–86
  recognize and analyze cues, 84
  risk factors, 84
Hypertensive emergency, 83f, 84
Hypertensive urgency, 83f, 84
Hyperthyroidism
  complications, 6
  definition, 6
  medical management, 6
  nursing management, 6–7
  recognize and analyze cues, 6
  symptoms, 5f
Hypoadrenalism. See Addison disease
Hypoglycemia, 10, 12, 14, 20, 124
  definition, 24
  medical management, 24
  nursing management, 24–25
  recognize and analyze cues, 24
  risk factors, 24
  symptoms, 23f
Hypothyroidism
  clinical manifestations, 7f
  complications, 8
  definition, 8
  medical management, 8
  nursing management, 8–9
  recognize and analyze cues, 8
  risk factors, 8

Hypothyroidism (Continued)
  symptoms, 7f
Hypovolemic shock, 92
Hypoxia
  assessment, 51f
  clinical signs and symptoms, 51f
  complications, 52
  definition, 52
  medical management, 52
  nursing management, 52–54
  recognize and analyze cues, 52
  risk factors, 51f, 52

· I ·

ICD. See Internal cardioverter-
    defibrillator
ICS. See Inhaled corticosteroids
IICP. See Increase in intracranial
    pressure
Ileal conduit/loop, 216
Ileitis. See Crohn's disease
Ileostomy, 116
Immediate triage, 246
Impaction, bowel elimination, 106
Impaired acetylcholine receptors,
    170
Impaired awareness, 146
Incontinence, bowel elimination, 106
Incontinent urinary diversions, 216
  ileal conduit/loop, 216
  nephrostomy, 216
  ureterostomy, 216

Increase in intracranial pressure (IICP)
    complications, 142
    Cushing triad signs. *See* Cushing triad
    definition, 142
    medical management, 142
    nursing management, 142–144
    recognize and analyze cues, 142
    risk factors, 142
    signs and symptoms, 141*f*
Inhalation therapy, 56
Inhaled corticosteroids (ICS), 54
Insulin, 14, 18
    deficiency, 10
Insulin resistance syndrome. *See*
        Metabolic syndrome
Intensive care unit, 142–144
Internal cardioverter-defibrillator (ICD),
        100
Internal fixation, fracture, 180
International Society of Hypertension, 80
Intestinal obstruction. *See* Bowel
        obstruction
Iron deficiency anemia, 36
Iron overload, delayed transfusion
        reactions, 41*f*, 42
Ischemic (occlusive) stroke, 150

–J–

Joint National Committee 8, 80
Joint replacements
    complications, 189*f*, 190
    definition, 190

Joint replacements *(Continued)*
    nursing implications, 190–192
    postoperative care
        total hip replacement, 190
        total knee replacement, 190–192
    preoperative care, 190

–K–

Keratoconus, 232
Keratoplasty. *See* Corneal transplant
        surgery
Kidney transplant rejection
    complications, 214
    definition, 214
    medical management, 214
    nursing management, 214–216
    recognize and analyze cues, 214
    signs and symptoms, 213*f*
Kock pouch, 116

–L–

Laparoscopic *versus* open
        cholecystectomy, 138
    complications, 138
    definition, 137*f*, 138
    nursing management, 138–140
Large intestine obstruction, 114
Latent TB infection, 68
LDL. *See* Low-density lipoprotein
Left CVA
    definition, 151*f*, 152

Left CVA *(Continued)*
  recognize and analyze cues,
    152–154
Left-sided heart failure, 98
  complications, 100
  definition, 100
  medical management, 100
  nursing management, 100–101
  recognize and analyze cues, 100
  risk factors, 100
  symptoms, 99f
Leukemia
  definition, 50
  medical management, 50
  nursing management, 50
  recognize and analyze cues, 50
  risk factors, 50
  symptoms, 49f
Lithotripsy, 206
Local governmental responsibilities,
    248
Lockjaw. *See* Tetanus
Lou Gehrig disease. *See* Amyotrophic
    lateral sclerosis
Low-density lipoprotein (LDL), 10
Lund-Browder chart, 218
Lung parenchyma, 56
Lyme disease
  complications, 220
  definition, 220
  medical management, 220
  nursing management, 220–221
  recognize and analyze cues, 220

Lyme disease *(Continued)*
  risk factors, 220
  symptoms, 219f

—M—

Management of DM
  definition, 18
  diet, 17f, 18–19
  exercise, 17f, 18
  medication, 17f, 18
  nursing management, 18–19
Man-made disasters, 242, 246
Mechanical obstruction, 114
Mechanical ventilation, 66, 72
Medication, diabetes management,
    17f, 18
Melanoma
  complications, 222
  definition, 222
  medical management, 222
  nursing management, 222–223
  recognize and analyze cues, 222
  risk factors, 222
  signs of, 221f
Menopause
  complications, 198
  definition, 198
  HAVOC, 197f
  medical management, 198
  nursing management, 198–199
  recognize and analyze cues, 198
  risk factors, 198

Metabolic syndrome, 11f
  complications, 28
  definition, 28
  features, 28
  healthy lifestyle, 28–29
  medical management, 28
  nursing management, 28–29
  recognize and analyze cues, 28
  risk factors, 28
  symptoms, 27f
Migraine headache symptoms
      (POUND)
  definition, 175f, 176
  medical management, 176
  nursing management, 176–178
  recognize and analyze cues, 176
  risk factors, 176
Mineralocorticoids, 30, 34
Minor triage, 246
Mixed hearing loss, 234
Multiple organ dysfunction syndrome
      (MODS), 72
Multiple sclerosis
  complications, 166
  definition, 166
  medical management, 166
  nursing management, 166–168
  recognize and analyze cues, 166
  risk factors, 166
  symptoms, 165f
Muscarinic receptors, 172
Myasthenia gravis
  complications, 170

Myasthenia gravis (Continued)
  definition, 170
  exacerbation risk factors, 170
  medical management, 170
  nursing management, 170–172
  recognize and analyze cues, 170
  symptoms, 169f
Myasthenic crisis, 170
Mycobacterium tuberculosis, 68
Myocardial infarction (MI)
  complications, 96
  definition, 96
  medical management, 96
  nursing management, 96–97
  recognize and analyze cues, 96
  risk factors, 96
  symptoms, 95f
Myocardial ischemia, 94
Myxedema coma, 8

–N–

National Response Framework,
      248
National Stroke Association, 150
Natural disasters, 242, 246
Nephrostomy, 216
Nephrotoxic injury, 208
Neurogenic (central) DI, 3f, 4
Neurogenic shock, 92
New York Heart Association (NYHA),
      98
Nicotinic receptors, 172

Noncardiogenic pulmonary edema.
    See Acute respiratory distress
    syndrome
Nonmechanical obstruction, 114
Non-ST-segment elevation myocardial
    infarction (NSTEMI), 96
Norepinephrine, 34
Normal elimination, bowel waste
    products
    definition, 106
    factors, 106
    POOPER and SCOOP, 105*f*
    problems, 106–108
Nosocomial pneumonia, 56
NSTEMI. *See* Non-ST-segment
    elevation myocardial infarction
Nutrition, 122, 210
NYHA. *See* New York Heart Association

–O–

Obstructive shock, 92
Obstructive sleep apnea
    complications, 74
    definition, 74
    medical management, 74
    nursing management, 74–75
    recognize and analyze cues, 74
    risk factors, 74
    symptoms, 73*f*
    treatments, 73*f*
Occlusive (ischemic) stroke, 150
Oculomotor nerve, 144

Office of Emergency Management, 248
Oliguric phase, 210
Open reduction, fracture, 180
Oral hypoglycemic therapy, 14
Organophosphate poisoning, 172
Orthostatic hypotension, 82
Orthotopic neobladder, 216
Osteoarthritis
    complications, 186
    definition, 186
    medical management, 186
    nursing implications, 186–188
    recognize and analyze cues, 186
    risk factors, 186
    symptoms, 185*f*
Osteomyelitis, 180
Osteoporosis
    definition, 192
    medical management, 193*f*, 194
    nursing implications, 194–196
    recognize and analyze cues, 192–194
    risk factors, 191*f*, 192
Ostomies
    definition, 116
    nursing management, 116–118
    pouching system, 116–118
    types, 115*f*

–P–

PACG. *See* Primary angle-closure
    glaucoma
PAD. *See* Peripheral arterial disease

Pancreatitis
   complications, 140
   definition, 140
   medical management, 140
   nursing management, 140
   recognize and analyze cues, 140
   risk factors, 140
   types, 139f
Papilledema, 144
Paraplegia, 158
Parasympathetic nervous systems, 172
Parkinson disease
   complications, 162
   definition, 162
   medical management, 162
   nursing management, 162–164
   recognize and analyze cues, 162
   risk factors, 162
   symptoms, 161f
Paroxysmal muscular contractions,
      178
PE. See Pulmonary embolism (PE)
Peptic ulcer disease (PUD)
   complications, 120
   definition, 120
   medical management, 120
   nursing management, 120–122
   recognize and analyze cues, 120
   risk factors, 119f, 120
Perimenopause, 198
Peripheral arterial disease (PAD), 86
Peripheral vascular disease (PVD), 218
   arterial versus venous ulcers, 85f

Peripheral vascular disease (PVD)
      (Continued)
   complications, 86
   definition, 86
   medical management, 86
   nursing management, 86–88
   recognize and analyze cues, 86
   risk factors, 86
Peripheral venous disease. See
      Peripheral vascular disease
Peritonitis
   complications, 110
   definition, 110
   medical management, 110
   nursing management, 110–112
   recognize and analyze cues, 110
   risk factors, 109f, 110
Phlebitis, 88
Pneumonia
   complications, 56
   definition, 56
   medical management, 56
   nursing management, 56–57
   recognize and analyze cues, 56
   risk factors, 56
   symptoms, 55f
Pneumothorax
   causes, 69f
   complications, 70
   definition, 70
   diagnosis, 69f
   medical management, 70
   nursing management, 70–71

Pneumothorax *(Continued)*
  recognize and analyze cues, 70
  risk factors, 70
  signs and symptoms, 69*f*
  treatment, 69*f*
POAG. *See* Primary open-angle
    glaucoma
Polydipsia, 4
Polyuria, 4
Postexposure prophylaxis (PEP), 178,
    240
Postictal seizures, 146
Post-mastectomy nursing care
  complications, 200
  definition, 199*f*, 200
  medical management, 200
  nursing management, 200–201
  recognize and analyze cues, 200
  risk factors, 200
Pre-exposure prophylaxis (PrEP), 240
Primary adrenal insufficiency. *See*
    Addison disease
Primary angle-closure glaucoma
    (PACG), 230
Primary intention, healing wounds,
    226
Primary open-angle glaucoma (POAG),
    230
Psychogenic nonepileptic seizures,
    146
Psychological stress, 244
PUD. *See* Peptic ulcer disease
Pulled muscle injury, 196

Pulmonary edema
  complications, 66
  definition, 66
  MAD DOG, 65*f*, 66
  medical management, 66
  nursing management, 66–67
  recognize and analyze cues, 66
  risk factors, 66
Pulmonary embolism (PE)
  complications, 64
  definition, 64
  medical management, 64
  nursing management, 64–65
  recognize and analyze cues, 64
  risk factors, 63*f*, 64
Pump failure. *See* Heart failure
PVD. *See* Peripheral vascular disease
Pyelonephritis, 203*f*, 204
Pyridostigmine, 172

–Q–

Quadriplegia, 158

–R–

Range of motion (ROM), 156
Recovery phase, 210
Red blood cell (RBC), 36
Renal calculi. *See* Urinary calculi
Renal replacement therapy (RRT), 210
Respiratory distress, 66
Respiratory failure, 8

Retained awareness, 146

Rheumatoid arthritis
definition, 188
medical management, 188
nursing implications, 188–190
recognize and analyze cues, 188
risk factors, 188
symptoms, 187*f*

Rickettsia rickettsia, 224

Right CVA
definition, 153*f*, 154
recognize and analyze cues,
154–156

Right-sided heart failure, 98
complications, 102
definition, 102
medical management, 102
nursing management, 102–103
recognize and analyze cues, 102
risk factors, 102
symptoms, 101*f*

Risk, injury, failure, loss, end-stage
kidney disease (RIFLE), 207*f*,
208

RMSF. *See* Rocky Mountain spotted
fever

Rocky Mountain spotted fever (RMSF)
complications, 224
definition, 224
medical management, 224
nursing management, 224–225
recognize and analyze cues, 224
symptoms, 223*f*

ROM. *See* Range of motion

RRT. *See* Renal replacement therapy

Rule of Nines, 218

–S–

Saffir-Simpson Hurricane Scale, 242

Sardonic smile, 178

SCI. *See* Spinal cord injury

Secondary intention, healing wounds,
226

Seizures
complications, 146
definition, 146
focal onset, 146
generalized onset, 146
medical management, 146–148
psychogenic nonepileptic, 146
recognize and analyze cues, 146
risk factors, 146
signs and symptoms, 145*f*

Self-esteem, 188

Self-management, 102

Senile cataracts, 228

Sensorineural hearing loss, 234

Septic (bacterial contamination)
acute transfusion reactions, 39*f*, 40
blood transfusion reaction, 44

Septic shock, 92

Sex hormones, 34

Shock
definition, 92
lung, 72

Shock *(Continued)*
  medical management, 92
  nursing management, 92
  recognize and analyze cues, 92
  septic, 92
  signs of, 91*f*
Short-acting β2-agonists (SABAs), 54, 58
Sickle cell disease/crisis, 36
  complications, 48
  definition, 48
  medical management, 48
  nursing management, 48–49
  recognize and analyze cues, 48
  risk factors, 48
  types, 47*f*
Simple partial seizures, 146
Sir hernia, 125*f. See also* Hernia
Skeletal traction, 184
  fracture, 180
Skin traction, 184
  fracture, 180
SLE. *See* Systemic lupus erythematous
Small intestine obstruction, 114
Spinal cord injury (SCI)
  complications, 158
  definition, 157*f*, 158
  medical management, 158
  nursing management, 158–160
  recognize and analyze cues, 158
  risk factors, 158
Spontaneous pneumothorax, 70

Sprains
  definition, 196
  medical management, 196
  nursing care, 195*f*
  nursing implications, 196
  recognize and analyze cues, 196
  risk factors, 196
State governmental responsibilities, 248
ST-elevation myocardial infarction (STEMI), 96
Stereotactic pallidotomy, 162
Stoma, 116
Strains
  definition, 196
  medical management, 196
  nursing care, 195*f*
  nursing implications, 196
  recognize and analyze cues, 196
  risk factors, 196
Strangulation, signs of, 126
Stress ulcers, 119*f*, 120
Stroke
  definition, 148
  FAST. *See* FAST recognition of stroke
  medical management, 148–150
  recognize and analyze cues, 148
  risk factors, 148
  symptoms, 147*f*
Struvite, 206
Subarachnoid bleeding, 150
Substernal chest pain, 94

Superficial vein thrombosis (SVT), 88

Superior vena cava syndrome, 92

SVT. *See* Superficial vein thrombosis

Syndrome X. *See* Metabolic syndrome

Systemic lupus erythematous (SLE)

    complications, 238

    definition, 238

    medical management, 238

    nursing management, 238–239

    recognize and analyze cues, 238

    risk factors, 238

    symptoms, 237*f*

Systolic HF, 100

–T–

TACO. *See* Transfusion-associated circulatory overload

TA-GVHD. *See* Transfusion-associated graft-*versus*-host disease

Technological disasters, 242, 246

Tension pneumothorax, 70, 92

Tentorial herniation, 144

Tertiary intention, healing wounds, 226

Tetanic muscle contractions, 178

Tetanus

    complications, 178

    definition, 178

    medical management, 178

    nursing management, 178

    recognize and analyze cues, 178

    risk factors, 178

    symptoms, 177*f*

Tetraplegia, 158

Thrombotic stroke, 150

TIA. *See* Transient ischemic attack

TIPS. *See* Transjugular intrahepatic portal-systemic shunt

Tonic-clonic seizures, 146

Total hip replacement, 190

Total joint arthroplasty, 190

Total joint replacement. *See* Joint replacements

Total knee replacement, 190–192

Toxic diffuse goiter, 6

Traction, care of patient in

    definition, 183*f*, 184

    nursing implications, 184–186

    types of, 184

TRALI. *See* Transfusion-related acute lung injury

Tranexamic acid, 46

Transfusion-associated circulatory overload (TACO), 39*f*, 40, 44–45

Transfusion-associated graft-*versus*-host disease (TA-GVHD), 41*f*, 42

Transfusion-related acute lung injury (TRALI), 39*f*, 40, 44

Transient ischemic attack (TIA), 148

Transjugular intrahepatic portal-systemic shunt (TIPS), 128

Transplantation of kidney, 214

Transurethral resection of the prostate (TURP)

    complications, 201*f*

    definition, 202

Transurethral resection of the prostate
(TURP) (Continued)
medical management, 202
nursing management, 202
postoperative complications, 202
recognize and analyze cues, 202
risk factors, 202
Triage
complications, 246
deceased, 246
definition, 246
delayed, 246
immediate, 246
minor, 246
nursing management, 246–247
recognize and analyze cues, 246
risk factors, 246
types, 245f
Triglyceride level, 28
Trunk muscles, 178
Tuberculosis (TB)
complications, 68
definition, 68
diagnosis, 67f
medical management, 68
nursing management, 68–69
recognize and analyze cues,
68
risk factors, 68
symptoms, 67f
treatment, 67f
TURP. See Transurethral resection of
the prostate

Type 1 diabetes mellitus
acute complications, 10
chronic complications, 10
definition, 10
insulin, 18
medical management, 10
nursing management, 10–11
recognize and analyze cues, 10
risk factors, 10
signs and symptoms, 9f
Type 2 diabetes mellitus
antidiabetic drugs, 18
complications, 12
definition, 12
medical management, 12
metabolic syndrome, 11f
nursing management, 12–13
recognize and analyze cues, 12
risk factors, 12
signs and symptoms, 11f
Types of bowel obstruction, 113f, 114
complications, 114
definition, 114
mechanical, 114
nonmechanical, 114
recognize and analyze cues, 114–116
risk factors, 114

—U—

Ulcers
arterial versus venous, 85f
development, 120

Ulcers *(Continued)*
  duodenal, 119f, 120
  gastric, 119f, 120
  stress, 119f, 120
Uncal herniation, 144
Ureterostomy, 216
Uric acid, 206
Urinary calculi
  complications, 206
  definition, 206
  diagnosis, 205f
  medical management, 206
  nursing management, 206–208
  recognize and analyze cues, 206
  risk factors, 205f, 206
  symptoms, 205f
  types of, 206
Urinary diversion
  complications, 216
  definition, 210
  nursing management, 216
  recognize and analyze cues, 216
  risk factors, 216
  types, 215f
Urinary tract infection (UTI)
  catheter-associated, 204–206
  complications, 204
  definition, 204
  medical management, 204
  nursing management, 203f,
    204–206
  recognize and analyze cues, 204
  risk factors, 204

Urinary tract infection (UTI) *(Continued)*
Urolithiasis, 206
US Department of Homeland Security,
  248
UTI. *See* Urinary tract infection
Uvulopalatopharyngoplasty, 74

–V–

Vasomotor symptoms, menopause,
  198
Vector-borne disease, 220
Venous leg ulcers, 86
Venous stasis (VS), 64, 88
Venous thromboembolism (VTE), 86
  complications, 88
  definition, 88
  medical management, 88
  nursing management, 88–90
  recognize and analyze cues, 88
  risk factors, 87f, 88
Vitamin B$_{12}$ deficiency anemia, 36
Vitamin D supplements, 194
VS. *See* Venous stasis
VTE. *See* Venous thromboembolism

–W–

Waist circumference, 28
Weather forecasters, 242
Weight-bearing exercise, 194
White lung, 72
Wound healing. *See* Healing wounds